LEARNING TO

DISCOVERING WEIGHT WASN'T

TAKE

ALL I NEEDED TO LOSE AND

CARE

HEALTH WASN'T ALL I STOOD TO GAIN

OF ME

Charity Bradshaw

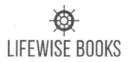

LIFEWISE BOOKS

LEARNING TO TAKE CARE OF ME

Discovering Weight Wasn't All I Needed to Lose and Health Wasn't All I Stood to Gain

Charity Bradshaw

The information in this book is the author's opinion and does not constitute medical advice. The content of this book is for informational purposes only and is not intended to diagnose, treat, cure, or prevent any condition or disease. Please seek advice from your healthcare provider for your personal health concerns prior to taking healthcare advice from this book.

Published by:

⊗ LIFEWISE BOOKS

PO BOX 1072
Pinehurst, TX 77362
LifeWiseBooks.com

To contact the author: CharityBradshaw.com

ISBN 978-1-958820-42-1 (print)
ISBN 978-1-958820-43-8 (ebook)

DEDICATION

To the broken but incredibly strong woman who
began this journey years ago with only a speck of hope—
Thank you for trying one more time.

WITH MY DEEPEST GRATITUDE,
I would like to thank:

My loving and supportive husband, Ted, who accepts me unconditionally, wants what's best for me, believes in my dreams, and stands by my side.

My children, who I want to be around for as long as I can.

My mom, who was my first fan and is my ultimate cheerleader.

My amazing friends who have encouraged me.

My brilliant team at LifeWise Books.

Day One or One Day—you decide.

UNKNOWN

CONTENTS

Start where you are.
Use what you have.
Do what you can.

ARTHUR ASHE

START HERE

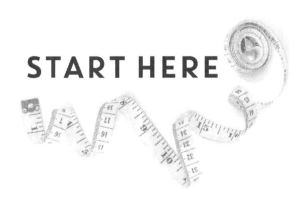

Life is hard and can certainly be unfair, but despite it all, I had to learn some very important things to achieve the freedom I wanted and shed the stuff holding me back. Stuff like limiting beliefs, destructive habits, excuses, unforgiveness, dishonesty, denial, and more were things I let dictate my experiences for much of my first forty years. It took several "come to Jesus" moments, along with an honest look into what my mind was telling me, to see that I was the one standing in my own way, not everything else I tried to blame it on.

Of all the books I have written, this one has taken the longest, and much of that is because the pain I discuss in here has run deep for decades. Even though I am years away from my last "day one," the pain is still easily accessible, and recounting it triggered a lot of old behavior when I first started writing.

What I did my best to communicate in these pages are the directions my mind went, as it often guides the ship. Behavior changes when the mind changes. While you may be reading this to find out how I lost a lot of physical weight, you will discover it was only a symptom of the actual problem. This isn't a weight-loss book. It is a reckoning I had with the touchy subject of personal stewardship. Stewarding myself—my mind, my body, my spirit.

Stewardship means "the responsible overseeing and protection of something considered worth caring for and preserving."[1] What I and many others have likely experienced is that it is easy to neglect something (i.e., ourselves) that isn't considered worth caring for. It is easy to let something of low value go into disrepair. What isn't always easy is changing the way we "consider" something. This journey you are getting ready to read about was largely the process of me assigning value to myself.

Let me be clear I have always been the go-getter, excellent student, responsible person, achiever, and everything else that looked good academically and professionally, etc. From a full-ride scholarship to the number one salesperson nationwide for my department, I didn't think I had a low estimation of myself. I knew I was smart and could count on my work ethic to get me pretty much anywhere I wanted to go, except…

I couldn't understand how I had all this drive, discipline, and determination in what seemed like every area outside of food and my physical body. What was the disconnect? I knew how to accessorize, do my makeup and hair, along with wearing a lot of black clothes to distract from my size or create a smoke and mirrors effect, but at nearly every weight I weighed on all the yo-yo diets, I still didn't like me. In fact, I loathed myself. It was as if my feelings were tangled up slinkies, and I didn't have the patience or know-how to sort it out. It was easier to throw the mess around and believe I had no choice.

When all those tangles finally made it where I could barely move, the only choice was to do the work. The hard work. The digging, reflecting, changing kind of work. The pain of change was finally less than the pain of staying the same. The things I had to untangle (and am still working on untangling) extended back to some of my earliest memories, where most mindsets were forged. My guess is you might be reading this for some insight into yourself as well. I pray that while our stories may not be identical, you can take any illumination you get from here to help light your path and take your next right step.

Chapter One

As I was growing up, it was
made clear that the fat me
wasn't welcome, that a
thin person was expected
and awaited, and impatiently so.

ARABELLA WEIR

Chapter One
GROWING UP

I can't remember much prior to elementary age, as far as food routines go, but I do remember I was a picky eater. I didn't like almost everything, especially vegetables. I joke now and say I wouldn't be alive if it wasn't for peanut butter and jelly. I also remember being fascinated with microwaving a piece of American cheese until the edges kind of burned and eating that at least once or twice a day. Looking back, I can see patterns of fixating on one or two foods and not deviating much from them because my pallet was so narrow.

Our family ate the occasional iceberg lettuce salad, which I did like, but there was not much variety outside of that. At this age, I thought corn was a vegetable, and I was good with that one, but if it was green and especially if it was soggy—no, thank you. My parents relied on canned vegetables, and I could not stand the texture of them. Since my mom was never really taught cooking skills, it makes sense that canned vegetables were largely her go-to. Her mother, my maternal grandmother, was basically raised without a mother. My grandmother's mother died young of tuberculosis, so my grandmother didn't get much mothering or training. This lack of experience, combined with my grandmother being a poor, single mom of two for many years, translated into hardly any cooking skills being passed down to my mom as well.

My mom never lived on her own before marriage, so she was thrust into being a homemaker, while learning on the fly at twenty years old. No doubt, she did her best with the tools she had at the time. By the age of twenty-three, my parents welcomed me. I had them all to myself for nearly three years when my first sister arrived. Twenty months later, another sister came, and nineteen months after that, the final sister made her debut. Four girls in roughly six years made for a wild time at nearly any given moment.

PICK ONE

With four kids and two parents, life was busy. We kids each had our interests and talents, but because of the sheer number of us, we had to pick one to focus on. I remember playing the piano since age eight. I also remember two seasons of being on a neighborhood soccer team. I don't recall being a star player or naturally athletic. I'm pretty sure I was average at best. So when it came time to pick what to focus on, music was where I excelled and seemed the logical choice.

At first glance, this choice might not seem like a big deal, but in hindsight, it was a pivotal decision. Soccer was my only physical activity. We were not a very physically active family. We lived near a busy road and were surrounded by elderly neighbors. There were no nearby kids in our neighborhood, so tag, chase, street ball, or anything else that would get us running around wasn't an option. There was a church across the street from our house where we could ride our bikes in circles around their parking lot, but no challenge or competition from other kids pushed us.

Our house in Dallas was nice but happened to be right inside the edge of a not-so-great school district. Even today, the school scores are still horrible. There also were some safety concerns. For these and possibly other reasons, our parents enrolled us in a small Christian school that was K-6th grade. It was within walking distance from our house but not for most of my peers. It was sad not having friends who lived nearby.

I remember the lunches I made for myself were pretty amazing. Peanut butter and jelly with extra peanut butter and cheese puffs to stuff inside the sandwich for that perfect crunch. Dreamy. I looked forward to lunch. Of course, there was the red-headed kid named Michael who constantly made fun of my sandwich creation, but he was the one missing out. I'm pretty sure I ate a PB&J sandwich nearly every day. Some days, I would skip the bread and put the peanut butter and jelly in a bowl and call it "peanut butter and jelly stirred up." So creative.

NOTICING THE DIFFERENCES

I was already a little bit heavier by this time. I had no idea how much I weighed, but I could tell I didn't look like most of my peers. I couldn't run as fast, couldn't cross the monkey bars, and nearly always got picked last for recess soccer. I didn't know if I was doing something "wrong," so I didn't change anything, but these differences did come with some sadness that I couldn't be like my friends. I wanted to be like them so badly. They looked happy. They had cute outfits while I had to dress much older due to the sizes I needed being offered only in the women's plus stores at the time. In my young mind, it seemed like everything was going for the skinny kids. It was like they had an advantage I couldn't have.

At the start of my fifth-grade year, my parents noticed I was bored and not exactly challenged in school, so they met with the administration and had me sit for a test, which resulted in me skipping the fifth grade. I didn't even know you could do that or that this was the reason I was being tested before taking it. When I came back to class the next day and was moved into the sixth grade, there was some explaining to do to the other students. Thankfully, my teachers handled most of that.

I was nine and then turned ten years old in sixth grade. Even though I was young, I felt normal at this school, for the most part, because I had been there since first grade. People were used to me, and I was used to them, but this was all about to change as I was officially aging out of this school and needed to find a next step. After my sixth-grade graduation, where I was voted "Most Likely to Star in One Flew Over the Cuckoo's Nest as the Cuckoo," the search for a new school was in motion.

WEIGHT COUNSELOR

I don't know if it was because I mentioned my frustration or because my parents noticed my weight increasing, but at some point in these earlier school years, my parents had me meet with a "weight counselor." I'm not sure what her title or credentials were, but she was a small-framed woman, much older than me, likely much older than my parents, who looked like she never had a weight problem in her life. Of course, I never asked her. I assumed because she was so petite. I wondered how she could possibly understand anything I was going through.

Our meetings consisted of me weighing in and her asking me questions from a workbook I was supposed to be reading and implementing. I know now I didn't have the skill, maturity, or attention span to make those changes on my own at that age. I believe my parents had good intentions and knew this was out of their lane, but the help for overweight kids was very dismal then.

While I don't remember exactly the circumstances that caused me to end up in this office, I do remember her teaching me the most random things, like how I could get some scientific machine and miniature carbon cartridge and make my own bubbly, watered-down grape juice. Who would want that anyways? I am still unsure. My guess is she was trying to teach me healthy swaps for stuff I'm sure I told her I couldn't (read: didn't want to) live without.

I think I wanted to make changes, but it was almost impossible to be the only one doing it. I didn't want to make a different dinner, different breakfast, and, on top of that, skip dessert, unlike everyone else. My sisters and parents weren't changing anything, so why should I? I wanted to be free like them. I wanted to be included. I wanted to say yes to anything and everything I wanted whenever I wanted.

Free.

In control.

What a delusion.

What I see now as one of the bigger problems was that I didn't know how to *want* to change my eating habits. I wanted what everyone else wanted—to be able to eat anything and everything yet have a skinny and capable physique. I didn't even totally make the connection between what I ate and what I weighed. I knew my weight surprised my mom enough she thought to get me help. She battled her weight while I battled mine, yet not much changed in our kitchen at home. Needless to say, nothing changed, things only got worse where my weight was concerned.

When you are with yourself every day, it's hard to notice the subtle changes. Weight crept on and so did shame and insecurity. No one had to tell me to be embarrassed, it just happened. No one had to tell me to start hiding my body, I wanted to. I subconsciously decided to get attention in other ways like grades, art, and music—things that didn't depend on the scale or clothing size.

MIDDLE SCHOOL

I remember touring a couple of schools with my parents looking for my next option. One was an all-girls school, which felt a little too fancy for me. It had a boarding school option, its own natatorium, a beautiful campus, and distinct uniforms. I instantly felt like an imposter there—like I didn't belong. Plus, at this point in my life, boys were often easier to be friends with because they were less dramatic. I couldn't fathom being happy at a school where it was all drama, all the time.

My parents landed on a private, college preparatory, Christian school with a remarkable education program. It was so rigorous they assigned summer reading. I wanted to be ready for this new and much larger adventure called seventh grade, so I read the book as soon as summer break started. Bad idea. I forgot everything by the time the school year began.

Middle school is no joke for anyone, but transferring in as a new kid to a new school while being younger and overweight was extremely tough. Most of the students at this school had been there since kindergarten and knew each other well. I had to quickly adapt to this much higher level of learning as well as changing classrooms and having a locker.

This school had the typical plaid skirt uniforms, and thankfully, pleated navy shorts were one of my options. I remember noticing there was something different about me from nearly all the other girls in my class; I was bigger. My stomach, my hips, my legs, and my hair...all bigger. How were these girls so skinny? I studied them, watched what they ate, and compared it to what I ate. It seemed similar. How did they do it? *This isn't fair,* I thought.

To add to the noticeable size difference was the fact that I was two years or more younger than my classmates. This didn't sit well with a few. With some honest reflection, I was probably a lot to be around. I was different. I liked big earrings rather than the simple pearl studs or classic hoops many of the other girls wore. My bangs were something of a marvel. I had glasses and a retainer. Easy target.

And a target I was. Peers broke into my locker, leaving mean notes and various bodily fluids on a semi-regular basis. The guy whose locker was above me didn't think twice about dropping his football pads on me. Whoops! I couldn't seem to catch a break. I came home filled with anger and rejection, which I would take out on my sisters and parents. Slowly but surely, my bold, vivacious personality changed into a more timid, weak version of myself. I hated it. I hated being something else only to be tolerated and not ridiculed.

One thing, good and bad, was that our class (grade) had eighty-one people in it. There was nowhere to hide. There were not a lot of friend-group options. We didn't have the typical public school diversification that allows you to connect over interests. This was sink or swim with the choices I had. I was able to find a small group of girls who let me sit with them at lunch, and for them, I am so grateful. We ended up being friends through our high school years as well.

MAKING A CHANGE

Freshman year rolled around, and I desperately wanted to look like these skinny girls. I was finally old enough to go to the gym and do some workouts, even though I didn't know much about what I was doing. I understood the cardio equipment and would pump out thirty to forty minutes on the Stairmaster*, knowing I was pre-burning all the calories of what I wanted to eat. *This is a foolproof plan,* I thought. I felt the pump from climbing all those stairs and knew I was weeks away from looking and feeling like all the skinny girls. This was going to be my year.

From my newfound workout routine, I started gaining a splinter of confidence and decided, since I didn't have any recent team sports experience, I would join the track team, and that would be the big ticket to my physical and social transformation. I had my mom take me shopping for some biker shorts so I wouldn't die from chaffing. I was ready—or so I thought.

Being in athletics required after-school practices. This meant my parents had to come pick up my sisters at normal dismissal and "hang out" for the extra time while waiting for me to finish because we lived a solid thirty minutes away. They didn't say it bothered them or make me feel like it was a problem, but

I was aware enough to know it was a sacrifice. In my mind, I had put extra strain on my parents, which made me feel bad but also made me try my hardest to make it worth their time and energy.

The first practice was finally upon us. I was so nervous I went to the bathroom several times before it even began. I walked over to the track and started awkwardly stretching, trying to copy what I saw everyone else doing because I had no clue what to do. The track coach was intimidating. At the time, he was the strength and conditioning coach for the Dallas Mavericks, the city's NBA team, and looked a little like Arnold Schwarzenegger. He was a winner and liked to coach winners.

I came into this practice hoping, praying, and believing it would help me change my life, change my body, and change my status. It did; however, I should have been more specific. Let's start with the warm-up that nearly killed me. I had no idea that the first thing we would do to get "warmed up" would be the hardest thing I'd ever done in my life. He had us form a single-file line and start running around the track. Then, the last person in line must sprint to become the first person in line while we were all STILL RUNNING.

What in the world?

I can't breathe.

My heart is pounding so hard.

Is this what dying feels like?

How is everyone else doing this so effortlessly?

Why does the coach hate us?

I don't remember much from the rest of that day. I only remember thinking that warm-up might kill me. I felt defeated, less-than, hopeless, and that my career as a freshman track runner might be short. Somehow, I convinced myself to show up the next day and the next for practice, but something was trying to get my attention.

One day before practice started, I went into the coach's office area to tell him about this horrible pain in my shins. It was excruciating. It felt like my shin muscles were so tight and sore they would snap my shin bones. I had seen some runners come out of this office with tape on various parts of their feet and ankles; perhaps, I needed to be taped. Maybe he was going to tell me I fractured my shins? I had been working hard, giving this my absolute all and then some.

"Excuse me, Coach," I said, trying to get his attention even after being in the office for almost a minute without acknowledgment.

"Yes, what do you need, uh...?" he said, trying to guess who I was.

"Charity." I let him off the hook since he clearly didn't know my name.

I said, "My shins are hurting very bad. I'm not sure what I did, but I can barely walk."

He said, "You have shin splints."

I waited for more information, guidance, treatment, or suggestions, and all I got was a visual of the top of his head as he was already focused back on the paperwork on his desk.

I said, "What do I need to do to get better? I can barely walk, much less run for practice."

He sat back, rubbed his eyes, and let out an annoyed huff of all the air he had, then stood up and walked over to me and said, "You should quit."

I was shocked. I hadn't planned on quitting. I wanted a path to recovery and to keep trying. This was the only sport offered by my school that I had any shot at, and I had only been on the practice roster for about a week. How could quitting possibly be his advice?

I questioned his suggestion and was met with him saying, "There are two things I can't stand: freshmen and girls."

My then thirteen-year-old brain couldn't believe what I was hearing, and my now adult brain is still infuriated. As any teen would, I began arguing that he wasn't even giving me a chance and had already marginalized and dismissed me mentally because I was, in fact, both a freshman and a girl.

I tried to answer him with any shred of medical knowledge I had about what could possibly be done to help my shins so I could stay on the team, to which he answered, "Look, I have forgotten more than you will ever know about fitness and training."

I was done.

Even if my shins could have improved fast enough to continue training, I knew I didn't want to be anywhere near this pig. My high school athletic career ended that day. I was relegated to P.E. with the rest of those who either couldn't make the cut or didn't want to. I was embarrassed, frustrated, still out of shape, and overweight, with no hopes of that changing anytime soon.

Athletics was a "have" or "have not" space in the school. There was no onramp or transitional plan for those on the outside looking in with hopes to one day be a part. Having children of my own now, it seems some of this mentality is still deeply ingrained in our society.

The individuals this misogynistic coach wanted to have around were career athletes requiring little to no effort on his part, athletes who would make his star shine brighter while he sat by and drank egg whites. I nor anyone like me at the time fit that mold; therefore, we didn't get the chance to experience the joy and satisfaction of the team sports he coached.

SOPHOMORE YEAR TRANSFORMATION

One of the first times I remember deciding to lose weight was at age thirteen, between my freshman and sophomore year. My mom was trying Nutrisystem', so I thought I would too. It was prepackaged, science food that gave the appearance of normalcy and fun with fewer calories. I thought if fewer calories were good, skipping a meal here and there must be even better.

I gave it a solid go and followed the all-or-nothing mentality. I was consistent. I didn't cheat once. I remember eating carrot sticks and light ranch dressing I brought to a birthday pool party while everyone else ate the cake. I had goals and believed suffering was the only way to get there. I was in food jail because I had been "bad" for so long. I had to pay for my food crimes one carrot stick at a time.

That summer, I lost a lot of weight through what felt like sheer torture and slight starvation. I looked incredible, even though I couldn't "see" it. I got down to a size six with no prior memory of ever being that small. I didn't like many pictures to be taken of me, especially if they showed my tummy area or legs. I remember my dad insisting I take a picture. He was proud of me. Yet, even at a six, I still felt big and thought I looked that way as well.

I went back to school that fall totally transformed (or so I thought) at the top of my game and the lowest of sizes. I relocated to the popular kids' tables and ditched my solid friends in hopes of climbing the social ladder with my new look. (To even write this is embarrassing. I don't know who I thought I was, but I ended up being a jerk face.) I got invited to a few cool kids' parties and knew my life was turning around.

My mindset was "goal achieved," as if this weight was simply a destination I arrived at rather than a perpetual practice requiring maintenance. This lack of understanding took me right back to my old eating habits. It should come as no surprise that the pounds I lost came back effortlessly, along with a few more, because I didn't maintain the methods that got me to that weight. Yet, I was surprised.

How could I have lost all that progress so easily? What took months to lose sure didn't take months to gain. Why was this so hard? My thirteen-year-old brain wasn't making the connection, and there was no internet to ask questions to and get ALL. THE. ANSWERS. This was the slipperiest of slopes, and I was sliding fast without anything to grab hold of.

Along with my vision of changing social statuses went my hopes of a Cinderella story with athletics as well. I thought I could prove "someone" wrong and have a solid "in your face" moment when all I proved was I was still weak, undisciplined, and disgusting. Those were a few of the toxic thoughts I was already sure of.

I was the loudest critic in my head, and I was hurtful. No mercy. No empathy. Just harsh judgment. Eventually, I tucked my tail and remorsefully crawled back to my true friends, who graciously took me in again.

Why was physical appearance of such a high value to the elusive popular crowd? Where was the "what's on the inside is what counts" card I could use to get myself some social cred? It felt like people wouldn't even try to get to know me simply because of what I looked like. They couldn't be seen talking to me or especially being nice to me. I somehow lowered their rank.

Once again, I toned down my boisterous personality and replaced it with what I thought was appropriate—shame and public shyness. I hated this version of myself because it wasn't who I was. Yet, I felt trapped by some unwritten social norm that said fat kids (especially girls) shouldn't get attention or try to get noticed. We should fade into the background since we are embarrassing. At least fat guys could go out for the football team and be linemen. There wasn't a hole deep enough to crawl in and hide.

Chapter Two

Shame corrodes the very
part of us that believes
we are capable of change.

BRENÉ BROWN

Chapter Two
COMPARISON, DENIAL, AND SHAME

ONE OF THESE THINGS IS NOT LIKE THE OTHERS

With four girls in our family, comparison seemed inevitable. We each had our thing, our talent, or what I saw as a superpower. For one of my sisters, her superpower (to me) was that she was skinny. I was very jealous of her. She seemed to have our dad's approval and pride more than the rest of us in the physical appearance arena. It didn't make sense to me. We had the same parents and gene pool, yet she got lucky.

This wasn't fair. She was able to wear all the cute clothes with no issue. She was our mom's Barbie® doll while I was stuck with plus-sized women's wear that was so serious and boring. The fashion world hadn't yet caught on that young girls could be plus sized too. I ended up having to dress decades older than I was including shoulder pads, mid-calf length skirts, pantsuits, and more.

Combine all that with my above-average intelligence and height and most people thought I was older than I was, resulting in me not fitting in anywhere. Even at church, our punishingly small youth group had an alpha female who made life miserable for anyone who didn't fall in line. My response ebbed and flowed as did my need for her approval. There were times I dished back plenty of attitude, but that always came with backlash from her and sometimes her mother.

Most of the time, it was easier to separate myself, sit alone, and try to focus on learning and moving forward than to get too distracted by what was happening. I tried telling myself I was taking the high road, but I was lonely, very lonely. I had no sense of belonging and no true community. This stage lasted for most of high school.

I watched my sister have boys chase her, date her, like her, and buy stuff for her while I was begging for a look. I remember wanting to go to homecoming so badly my freshman year that I had my youth group pray for me to get a date. One of my fellow youth group members offered to take me as a friend, and I cried as that was the nicest thing anyone had ever done for me.

Sadly, my parents felt I was too young to go to the dance, but they did allow him to go to the homecoming football game with me. I bought myself a mum and wore it with pride. I had a "date." Standing next to my friend during the game made me feel very special. Outside of this incident, there were no other dates, true boyfriends, or noble pursuits to speak of.

There was the occasional boy with ulterior motives who didn't want to be public about things. They probably learned quickly that girls with low self-esteem are the perfect targets for this kind of agenda. Many times, we will do anything for attention or connection in hopes that a relationship will bud even from this kind of crappy start.

CHEESE FIXES EVERYTHING

Lowering my standards was something I had become well acquainted with. Having little to no feeling of intrinsic worth made it easy to be used. I would rather have had something over nothing. This "using" further ingrained the message that I was of low value, my feelings didn't matter, and I wasn't worth taking good care of or, God forbid, treasuring. Taking care of myself seemed pointless (not that I thought of it that way as a kid). What was appealing was soothing or rewarding myself with food to ease the pain and fill the time.

I had a hard day. *Have some ice cream.*

Today was super stressful. *Some fries will go perfect with that.*

I felt a lot of negative feelings. *Chocolate.*

Loneliness sucks. *Cheese fixes everything.*

Rather than feeling the feelings or releasing the pain, I fed them. All of them. I was already embarrassed, so why not self-medicate with food? Recently, I heard a registered dietician say something like, "If hunger isn't the problem, food isn't the solution." What I would give to have that insight all those years ago.

Food seemed to have all the answers. It made the angry voices go away, the loneliness be not so noticeable, and the sting of rejection seem a little more bearable. It was like a happy pill in the moment that came with a huge side effect of shame. I didn't fully put together that my eating behavior was emboldening a loud and nasty voice of self-hatred for my physical condition. I was making the problem I hated worse. It was a vicious cycle.

Feel shame.

Eat.

Feel shame for eating.

Eat more.

Feel shame for how I look.

Eat.

Feel shame for eating…

If you're reading this book, you likely know exactly what I'm talking about and are well acquainted with the thoughts of, *Why do I keep doing this? Why can't I stop? What is my problem? Everyone else has it under control. I am disgusting.* Try being left alone with that voice for an hour, a day, a week, or a year. I never wanted to be left alone with myself.

I came to the (easy way out) conclusion that being overweight was my lot in life. It was how things were, and I had no control over that. The women in my family seemed to run large, so no wonder I did too. Why try to fight it? Why not give in and let it be? I was "big boned," tall, and built to survive a famine, was the story I told myself. But did I believe it at my core? No. I had no other explanation in my teenage mind as to why I couldn't lose and keep off weight. It couldn't possibly be my fault.

I finished high school no healthier than I started. I did begin my inner revolution around my senior year when I started to care a little less about what others thought and began finding my voice again. One big step I took was when there was an opening for our school mascot my senior year, I decided to try out and got it. While this didn't change my status, I made tons of memories and enjoyed a small slice of being on the pep team.

COLLEGE

At the age of sixteen, I graduated and was offered an art scholarship to Southern Methodist University (SMU). Because I was so young, my parents had me commute rather than stay on campus. I got a part-time job and was taking eighteen hours my first year. I would pack my lunch most days and head to the campus commuter lounge. This was not the social mecca at all. We had one television that a middle-aged woman controlled because she had to watch her soaps every day.

This lounge was also where the campus burger and fries restaurant was located. There were days I would polish off the lunch I brought and then rationalize a large order of fries on top. I wasn't hungry; the impetus was environmental. I never thought to eat anywhere else because there wasn't anywhere else to go. The "freshman fifteen" was in full effect and maybe a few more.

I quickly realized how expensive SMU was and that it wasn't going to be sustainable for three more years. After my freshman year was over, I transitioned to our local community college and had a great second year. Everyone was a commuter, so I was just like everyone else. One thing led to another, and I ended up auditioning for a vocal group that welcomed me my second semester there. I joined and received a scholarship to cover private voice lessons.

Before completing my second year, which was when most wrapped up their time at community college, I applied to Oral Roberts University (ORU) and was accepted. Knowing neither I nor my family could swing private school tuition, I also applied to an outside organization for a potential full scholarship to ORU. They awarded this then $40K scholarship to one guy and one girl each year. After a grueling application process, I waited and waited, hoping to hear back in time to make plans.

One glorious day while working my retail job, my parents called to let me know I was the female recipient for that year. I couldn't believe it. All that hard work academically was paying off. This was my chance at a fresh start and new major—music! I was going to go and be myself without any apologies, but I wanted to look as good as I could going in.

Per usual, the diet industry was churning out product after product, promising results and all the happiness that went with them. In the 1990s, fen-phen™ (a combination of fenfluramine and phentermine) was the newest craze. My mom tried it, so of course, I tried it. I didn't let anyone else know I was taking it as needing a pill to lose weight was also shameful.

I was in the first year of my music degree and loved how awake and alert I felt while not feeling hungry. I was not sure what my weight was, but I knew I was losing it and becoming more awesome by the day. One morning, I was in music history class and felt like my heart was beating out of my chest. I was twitchy, and the room appeared a little blurry. I was terrified I would die of a heart attack or some sort of episode simply because I wanted to lose weight so bad I was taking pills.

Sadly, that episode scared me so much that it ended my "awesome" streak, as those side effects were too much to tolerate. I was bummed that this magic pill couldn't work for me. After all, this was college, and another "freshman fifteen" was en route. Every meal was served buffet style in the cafeteria, and my optimal health was never a thought as I entered the blissful oasis of endless food.

Plate of fries? Sure.

Four to six freshly baked chocolate chip cookies with lunch? Heck yeah.

Any ounce of restraint I may have had fled right out as I walked in the door. This was the highlight of my day nearly three times a day. Every meal was a reward or an escape. An escape from the emptiness of not having a boyfriend or significant other. A reward for how stressful school was. For all the things—it muted the voices for those fleeting minutes and numbed the pain. It literally made me feel happy while I was eating. I needed it.

DENIAL

I don't know if it was one of the chapel services or a Bible study I went to, but there was talk about battling addiction. No one ever mentioned food as an addiction, but that notion flashed inside my head. Maybe it was God trying to gently get my attention and bring awareness, but I wasn't ready to be *that* honest yet. I was as serious about food as an addict about their next hit, but I was sure I was not addicted. *How can you even be addicted to food? You need food to survive.* The term "addiction" is only used when something is illegal or illicit, right? Food was everywhere. I had access to it pretty much all hours of the day, between what was in the cafeteria and the stash I had in my room.

I was NOT an addict, and I was determined to prove it. I went so far as to check out Food Addicts in Recovery Anonymous to confirm my lofty and denialist opinion. I was absolutely offended at what I found out. As part of "recovery," they expected people to weigh and measure their food, cut out all flour and sugar, not eat between meals, and avoid individual binge foods. That was unrealistic and torturous. They might as well put someone in food jail and pass the obscure gray sludge you see in movie prison scenes.

No, thank you.

Here came my internal arguments (a.k.a. tantrums) and skewed logic (skewed on purpose because who wants to acknowledge they are an addict):

- Who in this world we live in could figure out how to eat without flour and sugar? They are in everything. *(Everything delicious.)*

- What if I was hungry in between meals, should I STARVE? *(Insert a near fainting expression.)*

- Binging is something you do only if you're going to make yourself puke, and I hate puking, so I must not have any binge foods. *(Note to self: don't look up what binging means.)*

- Weighing and measuring my food? That sounds like perfectionism, and I am NOT okay with that. *(I don't want accountability.)*

- They are trying to control me and force me to eat foods I don't like. They are bad, and I need to be safe. *(I must be in control, so I can keep eating what I want when I want it.)*

As much as I wish I could have unknown everything I read about food addiction, I couldn't. But I pretended I did and went about business as usual.

REQUIRED HEALTH
AND PHYSICAL EDUCATION CLASSES

One thing I appreciate about my time at ORU was they required a health and fitness class every semester as well as a fitness test of a timed three-mile run, walk, or swim version. They believe we are more than our brains. We are spirit, mind, and body. A daily investment in the physical body is an important and critical part of a holistic education. I was sure I would not pass the fitness test because I wasn't a fast walker, and running wasn't a thing due to all the extra pounds. But I was willing to give it a try.

There were plenty of choices from cardio classes, golf, bowling, and conditioning. I decided to take the conditioning class first to try and help me build up to the three-mile fit test. The very first session of that class, the instructor asked us to write down on a card how many times a day we pooped. *(Am I in the right class?)* No joke. She passed out note cards, and we had to write our names and how many times. This was awkward for all of us at first, but then she explained her story of being a colon cancer survivor and the importance of regularity and how that plays into our overall health. No one ever talked about this.

As a survivor, I was blown away by how vibrant, healthy, and positive she was. She didn't sugarcoat things she was teaching us but was armed with grace and true love for her students. In her class, I learned some foundational things about health, food, and fitness but wasn't ready to tiptoe into the salad bar in the cafeteria yet. The seeds were planted though, and for that, I am grateful. I took my first fitness test and made a C, which was no surprise. I was thankful I didn't fail and had a solid benchmark to beat in the following semesters.

My personal favorite athletics class had to be badminton. I was decently good at it, and the coach was great about matching us with other students at our skill level. I took that class for a year (the school's max number of times) and then took advanced badminton the following year. If there was ever to be a wall of photos for badminton legends, I think my picture would have ended up there.

Physical activity was never a challenging issue for me. I love moving and am highly competitive. There were many things I "missed" out on because I didn't have the speed or agility that being a less-obese version of myself would have allowed me to participate in. I do have some regrets about that. Who am I kidding? Lots of regrets.

AN HONEST FRIEND

One of the benefits of home being only a four-hour drive away from college was I could easily visit for holidays. I would often find a few friends who couldn't get to their homes and invite them out so they wouldn't have to stay on a virtually empty campus. Thanksgiving of my junior year rolled around, and about four friends didn't have a way to get home, so we made the drive in two cars to my house in Dallas. I had three friends in my car, and my friend Calvin followed in his.

Calvin was a guitarist in the band I formed and had a few friends in Dallas that he visited while staying with us. One night, he was out kind of late seeing them, and I told my parents I would wait up and let him in. There were no cell phones back then, so I had to be patient and wait without communication.

He finally returned to a quiet house where I had only one small light on in the living room. I asked him how his time with his friends went and so forth, which eventually turned into a discussion that changed my life. While we were talking, he began looking at some of the pictures on the walls and noticed a younger me in the photos. The conversation was still about him and maybe some broad life concepts at the time. Then what felt like suddenly, he basically asked me why I was overweight.

He said something to the effect of, "You're a talented musician. Do you want to go somewhere with your music? Don't you think your weight will affect that?"

I was dumbfounded.

What a question? What nerve?

He talked about how in the pictures of when I was a child, I wasn't as overweight and asked about what changed. I don't remember if I cried at that moment, but I felt very exposed. This wasn't something you talk about or "call out," especially about a girl. How could he?

He went on to explain how much he truly cared for me and was willing to risk our friendship to help me see that my weight would be a hindrance, not only to my health but my future.

Most of that fell on deaf ears at the time because the truth hurt. I armored up and told him that was a rude thing to say to someone who invited him into their home. He offered to leave and drive back to campus, but I didn't want to have to explain that to everyone else, so I told him not to worry about it.

I cried myself to sleep that night. The voices of shame, regret, self-hatred, and loneliness were ringing in my head. We went back to school, and I tried to forget about the whole thing.

SPRING FLING

Spring break rolled around, and a group of good friends invited me to go to Colorado to go skiing. I had never been to Colorado or skiing, so this was an incredible opportunity. One of the guys from my band was also on the trip and was a beginner like me. We were the only two rookies from our group and ended up spending a lot of time together on the bunny trails. The trip concluded with us driving back and adding a stop in Dallas.

While driving to Dallas, this guy asked me to be his girlfriend. I did not see this coming at all. We were in a band and goofed a lot, but until he asked, I had only seen him as a friend. I was swept off my feet. I hadn't had a proper or public boyfriend in college, and this was exactly what my self-esteem needed. I told him I would love to be his girlfriend. We didn't share the news with the rest of the group yet, but I was beaming from the inside out. I couldn't wait to tell everyone because I was so excited. I wanted that validation and status.

I was "wanted."

I was "desired."

I was "attractive."

I was "enough."

At that time, it seemed those things were only true if felt by someone else for me first.

We began sharing our news with friends and family, and it was fun having someone to meet for meals in the cafeteria as well as walk to classes with. Towards the end of the semester, we had a conversation where he asked me if I thought we were together for more than merely boyfriend and girlfriend. I wasn't sure exactly what he meant, so I had him clarify. He talked about a more long-term thing, like marriage.

Oh my gosh! Did I just get a proposal over nachos at Taco Cabana? I told him I would very much like that.

I AM NOT GOING TO BE ALONE!!!!!—was the thought going through my head. I was going to be married. I was going to be a wife. My future could be planned out now. I don't have to be ashamed anymore. Someone wants me. I am acceptable. Having someone love me made me feel beautiful. I came out of my shell even more. I was happy. I was smiling all the time. I loved this new me.

There wasn't a ring at the time as it was so spontaneous, but we were engaged. I called home so proud of myself. I had found a husband. His home was about thirty minutes away from my home, which made it even more "meant to be." We were going to be able to see each other over the summer. This was perfect. We even planned an outreach concert for our band. Everything was falling into place—until it wasn't.

At about midnight on Father's Day morning, he called to break up with me and told me not to try to get back together with him. This was out of nowhere. His dad's health was failing, and my only rationale at that time was he was feeling conflicted about how he spent the time he had left with him. I was humiliated, devastated, and alone again.

This grief was palpable. My mom would listen and do her best to console me as I mentally watched the future I had envisioned crumble and fade. I did what many women do when they break up with someone—chopped my long hair off. And like many of those women, I quickly regretted that decision as well. However, the next series of choices were much better.

I decided to start exercising and eating better. I was going to return for my senior year different—better, skinnier. If he was going to see me again, he was going to wish he had never broken up with me. I lost about twenty-five pounds in the remaining summer months and was excited to return to campus. What I forgot to plan for was having to tell every person who knew us about the breakup. It got old really quick. Everyone assumed we were still together and were asking about us. It rubbed the wound raw again. Thankfully, after a few short weeks, he started dating someone else and quickly announced they were getting married, so the questions stopped.

SENIOR YEAR

My final year in college was wonderful. I was more comfortable in my skin; I had great friends and a close dorm family. I continued exercising while making only minimal changes in the food department. One focus was only drinking water, not a glass of water, but four to five glasses per mealtime. I proudly lined the front of my tray with these cups and did my best to drink them every time. If I had any water left over, I would pour it on any food remaining on my plate so I wouldn't graze while chatting after I was satisfied or full. I can't take credit for this idea, though. I saw another girl doing it and thought it was a brilliant tool to add to my tool belt.

I wish I could go back and tell myself how much I should appreciate every little change I made. I would also tell myself my body never looked as bad as I thought, so stop hating it. So much energy was wasted using negative messages to try to motivate or change myself. I see this now but didn't see it then and would probably tell myself this too.

PANIC AT THE DISCO

While I was excited to be nearing the end of college, I was also nervous. I had a great life, great friends, and even a successful side hustle of doing hair and makeup to help pay for my car. But there was something looming over my head—*WHAT IN THE WORLD WILL I DO ONCE I GRADUATE?* I knew when I started my degree plan the chances of me going into music post-graduation were slim to none. I studied music because I loved it and enjoyed the cultural experience of it. I had no clue of the path I was going to take after they handed me my diploma.

One Friday night in the fall semester, I was in my dorm room getting ready to go to an all-skate event our college sponsored when I started hyperventilating. I didn't know if it was the onset of an asthma attack, but my hands and lips began to tighten, and I was freaking out. I called home, and my parents talked me down out of what I know now was a panic attack. Panic attacks were not discussed or really generally known about back then. I realized my mind had a lot of questions and very few answers, which caused me to sort of short-circuit. It felt like I was in a permanent loop or hamster wheel with no signs of slowing down.

Not having answers didn't feel safe to me. I felt powerless and out of control, two of my least favorite feelings. I prided myself on knowing what the next step was going to be and how confident that made me look and feel. At this point, all I could see was a blurry haze. I translated this lack of vision into weakness and needed to eliminate it quickly. Here came more negative messages, negative energy, self-hatred, and disgust.

The wounded-beatdown me soothed the pain with food. I could control that. I could comfort myself that way because I "deserved it." I wish I had known then that I was only driving the knife deeper into myself by treating an emotional problem with a food solution. The only problem food is capable of solving is hunger. It pretty much makes every other problem worse. Then the cycle of feeling gross from being full, having a whacked-out blood sugar, to shame for eating like a pig, and having no self-respect or self-love began again.

Having all-access to food in college did not help this cycle. Occasionally, I would notice skinny girls and their habits and wonder how they could bypass the fries, cookies, chips, and soft-serve ice cream. *What willpower! What self-control!*

THEY were amazing.

I was not.

THEY were respectable.

I was not.

THEY were getting attention and boyfriends.

I was not.

As any person with a solidly bad relationship with food would do, I headed to the gym to punish those calories away. More time on the elliptical, heavier weights, more reps, and more pain, all in the attempt to "make sure I didn't eat that way again." What a crock. I knew I would, but somehow, this made me feel less disgusting.

Chapter Three

We work to feed our appetites;
Meanwhile our souls go hungry.

ECCLESIASTES 6:7[2]

LIFE AFTER COLLEGE

Chapter Three

PARTY LIKE IT'S 1999

May of 1999 came around, and sure enough, I graduated. I said goodbye to friends, packed my dorm room up for the last time, and drove home. I don't remember exactly how much of the drive was spent crying, but I know it was a good bit. Thankfully, my family had a gym membership, so I was able to jump right into working out again, and I quickly got a good job working for Nordstrom and was very successful at it.

With these two things in place, I created a decent routine for myself. If I had a later shift, I would work out first. If I had an early shift, I worked out after. Pretty simple. One thing I didn't notice for a while was that I was actually losing weight without thinking about it. Apparently, moving away from the all-you-can-eat cafeteria helped me drop about fifteen or so more pounds. Hallelu!

One late fall afternoon, while I was working at Nordstrom, my mom called to say there was a change in plans. That night we scheduled to have dinner with my dad after he arrived home from the airport. She told me to not worry about dinner and take my time at the gym and not rush home. I didn't have a good feeling about this call. My immediate thoughts were wondering what my dad had done because my mom sounded very serious. I went and sat down in the fitting room area and started crying.

One of my coworkers came over to see if I was alright, and I told her, "I think my parents are getting a divorce."

She said, "How do you know?"

I said, "I just have this feeling."

I couldn't get a grip on the crying. I would stop and then start right back up again. My manager was so kind to let me leave early, so I did what my mom suggested and spent a long time at the gym. By the time I got home, it was dark out. I parked in our driveway and opened the garage, only to find my parents still in the car talking. They waved me on to not disturb them. This did not bode well.

I went inside and crashed on my twin bed. My mind was running through all the possible scenarios of what happened, and I arrived at the same place every time—my dad cheated. I don't know how much time passed, but I didn't get up from my bed until my mom came in. She opened my door, and we looked at each other with pause.

I asked, "So, are you getting a divorce?"

She said, "Yes."

I asked, "Did Dad cheat on you?"

She said, "Yes."

I said, "I don't think you have the balls to do it."

She said, "I do, and I will."

Until now, my mom had been very subservient and lived as a doormat to him and several more dominant personalities. As a teen, I remember talking down to her because I didn't respect her based on how she let others treat her. I didn't think she was capable of being independent. She hadn't ever been on her own before. She went from living with her parents to being married and skipping the single life. She had a good job but couldn't support a house or household. How was she going to go through with this?

Slowly but surely, I brought my three younger sisters up to speed on the impending divorce. I couldn't bear that information on my own. I didn't have anyone to talk to in-depth. We each took the news in our own way. Some felt angry, some pretended nothing was wrong, but we all felt the only rug we knew ripped out from under us.

My mom moved into one of the auxiliary bedrooms while my dad stayed in their room. The divorce process took about three months. Our house, where I thought I would bring my kids to one day, was on the market to be sold for almost that entire time. Imagine living in a house with *both* divorcing parents while keeping your house show-ready for three months. It was torture. We did find some relief from the tension when my dad had work trips, but the eggshells we walked on returned as soon as he did.

MUST WORK OUT

The gym was where I spent most of my free time outside of work to dodge going home. I didn't yet have many (or really any) local friends yet, but because of my frequency at the gym, I started chatting with the club manager. She mentioned one day that she was going to start training for a fitness competition and asked if I wanted to train with her. I said I would do the exercise part, but no way was I going to do the whole flank steak and cucumber diet she had to do to get to such a low body fat towards the end.

We worked out twice a day, one hour of heavy strength training and the other of cardio. I was so strong. I wish I had a picture of myself because I'm sure I was crazy fit. I lost another seven pounds simply by changing my routine. This was the lowest weight I ever remember weighing as an adult, and I STILL THOUGHT I LOOKED FAT!

How is that possible? I will tell you how—body dysmorphia. That is a fancy term meaning, "a mental health disorder in which you can't stop thinking about one or more perceived defects or flaws in your appearance—a flaw that appears minor or can't be seen by others."[3]

Some of the symptoms of this disorder I experienced were:

- strong belief you have a defect that makes you ugly or deformed
- belief that others notice and make fun of or mock this defect
- trying to hide or mask the defect with clothing, makeup, or styling
- constantly comparing yourself to others
- frequently checking yourself in the mirror, over-grooming, and skin picking

This isn't something that only affects the overweight or obese. You will find it in every community from body builders to models. In fact, not all who are overweight or obese deal with dysmorphia. Some are content and even embrace their size for one reason or another. For me, it was relentless. Between all the mirrors around from working in retail and the gym, I was constantly reminded of everything wrong with me.

Despite being at my personal best weight, I still couldn't fit most of the clothes in the area I worked in. My clientele was nearly all skinny women who could walk into pretty much any store and find anything they wanted. Why can't I be like them? I was working so hard, but what they had was unattainable to me. I was somehow not special that way.

BAD CHOICE PARADE

Between my parents' divorce, the huge adjustment of graduating college, leaving my friends behind, not feeling good enough because of my size, and still not having a boyfriend, I started to spiral. I didn't know it, but I was in full-blown depression. At the time, mental health was not discussed, much less understood, and I was ashamed of my inability to pull myself together. I couldn't focus on anything positive. The self-hatred I had only worsened. There was even a period of six weeks where I didn't sleep at all. It made me hate being alone. I decided if I was going to be awake, I was going to be out.

Nothing was louder than being alone. If I was alone, the voice in my head was going to beat me up and leave me to die. It reminded me of how unlovable, disgusting, fat, unwanted, and less-than I was. It made me terrified to be alone. So I made sure to be alone as little as possible.

With this low view of myself, I was an easy target for guys who had less than noble intentions. I was ready to make some bad decisions in hopes of finding love and getting attention. If it was Latin Night at the club, I was there. If it was Ladies Night at the bar, I was there. If it was a karaoke cash contest, you know it—I was there. I even talked with guys online, and if they sounded interesting, I met them in public to hang out. I put myself in some precarious situations, some that could have led to horrible outcomes, but somehow, I managed to not totally self-destruct.

FINDING MY LOCAL TRIBE

One of the ways I met more people after returning home from college was through church. My parents were pastoring a small church up until around when I graduated, but there wasn't anyone my age there. They suggested I check out another local church known for having lots of singles in the mix. I started going and enjoyed the preaching as well as the social aspect. They were great at helping put people in the same age and relationship status together. For example, my group was singles, ages twenty-five to thirty-three. I was twenty-three at the time but was already working and out of college and didn't feel the college group was where I fit.

I began attending regularly and quickly found a small group (which was based on zip code) to hang out with. It didn't take long for that small group to outgrow the leader's house, so one of the guy members and I branched out and started our own to help accommodate the growth. I met several dear friends in this group. Everyone seemed to be going through difficulties and facing things we held deep inside, but we made our time together mostly fun instead of focusing on the drama or trauma.

My co-leader and I ran a successful small group for over a year. Our group continued to grow and so did the fun. I felt like I was having a positive impact on other people's lives, which distracted me from the mess I was inside. If I was busy, I didn't have time to think or feel, so I made sure the schedule was full. Work, gym, friends, going out, repeat.

During this time, there were many Sunday mornings I attended church with a hangover. My weekends usually started on Thursday nights and continued until the wee hours of Sunday morning. Every night wasn't off the rails, but since I wasn't sleeping, I wasn't usually home. Anything to delay or distract from the pain was part of my routine. Even one or two drinks allowed me to stop thinking about all my flaws for a while and tap into the courage I wish I had all the time. Despite knowing how low I would feel the next day, I didn't let that stop me from the bliss of a few hours of forgetting. Thankfully, I never went out alone. I usually had at least one or more friends alongside, and we would look out for each other.

A WEDDING IN LA JOLLA

Couples certainly formed out of our church small group, and some went on to get married. One of those couples asked me to be a bridesmaid as well as sing at their wedding. I was honored. I had never been in a wedding before, much less to the beautiful city of La Jolla, California. I went with the other bridesmaids to the dress shop where there were measurements taken but no dresses to try on. The bride had decided what she wanted for us, a near flesh tone pink, satin dress that would be difficult for nearly anyone to wear, much less someone who struggled with body issues.

My opinion wasn't asked for or wanted, so I kept it to myself. Several months went by from the fitting to when we received them, and when it came in, it didn't fit. I was mortified. There was no stretch or fabric to let out, and I didn't have enough time to order a new one, so I had to be what changed in this equation. I turned my workouts up a notch and did some tweaking on my diet to accommodate this truth-telling, unforgiving dress. I let it hang in my closet until the last minute before crazy tailoring would have to happen. Low and behold, by the time the wedding came around it fit with some extra room to spare.

When I accepted this invitation, I was in what felt like an "okay" place, but by the time the wedding rolled around, things had gotten darker. I didn't realize till I was in the thick of the ceremony that this was likely too soon for me to be at a wedding considering my parents' divorce was so fresh. As soon as the photos were finished, I made the most of the last ten minutes of the open bar before the reception began.

Thankfully (to me then), the alcohol didn't stop after the open bar. There was wine at dinner, and being at the wedding party table, they made sure our glasses were always full. Champagne toast? Yes, please. I couldn't feel anything. I almost couldn't stand up but was on the dance floor. I was about to leave and go to a club with a guy I just met from the wedding party when my friend, who attended the wedding with me, intercepted and drove me back to the hotel. I ugly cried the entire ride and eventually, cried myself to sleep. I was drowning.

A CLEAN SLATE

In late May of 2001, my roommate decided she was going to move back home for personal reasons. We were mid-lease, which meant I had to either pay the full amount for our townhome or find another roommate if I wanted to stay where I was. Between the lack of sleep, late nights, and mindless spending, I was coming to the end of myself. I was physically exhausted and felt gross from everything being all over the place. The idea of finding a new roommate sounded overwhelming, and while I could swing the full rent, that would have certainly put a dent in my fun money.

I decided to phone a friend who was like a brother to me. He and I met in college as music majors, were both pastor's kids, and had been there for each other through some very hard things. After getting a record deal, he and his brother moved to Nashville and were living there when not on tour. I explained my situation to him, and out of nowhere he said, "You should just move to Nashville..."

He kept on talking, but for me, everything became silent after that phrase. It was as if time stood still for a few seconds for me to process the thought. I had so many questions in such a short time. Why Nashville? I've never even been to Nashville, and I can't stand country music. Is this my Nineveh? Don't people need me here in Dallas? Leave my well-paying job and insurance? Move away from my family?

While my strategist brain went to work on all the reasons why I shouldn't go, my heart felt the deepest peace. I knew in my gut this was the right thing to do. The logical side of me still wanted to "confirm" this decision with a few people I trusted. I first asked my grandma what she thought. I knew she would say, "Don't go." To my surprise, she was in favor of the move and cheering me on. Next, I asked my mom, who I thought would question the idea. She thought it was great as well. Finally, I asked a longtime family friend, thinking he would have some concerns, and again, no.

They all were supportive of my move, which was both relieving and terrifying. At this point, I didn't have any excuses. No reasons to back out. Everyone was basically packing my bags for me. Once the shock of the idea wore off, the next thing that came to mind was this was an opportunity for me to start over—a clean slate. I could reinvent myself and leave out the stuff I didn't want to keep doing anymore and add the stuff I knew I should be doing.

This perspective gave me such excitement for the new adventure I was about to begin. I had roughly six months left on my current lease by the time I made the decision, which meant I was moving right around the beginning of the year. How perfect! New year, new beginning. I planned to use that time to save up money, find a job, and sign for an apartment.

Since my friend already lived in Nashville, I wouldn't be all alone in a new city. At least I had that going for me. He gave me some pointers on what areas were good to live in and some to avoid. I had an apartment locator find a place with all the amenities I wanted and booked a trip for mid-November to scope it out. At this time, the trip was still a few months away.

ANOTHER WAVE CRASHED

One of my friends from our small group invited me on a quick two-day trip to Vegas using his points, and within a few hours, I was packed and ready to go. In traditional Vegas-style, the drinking started at the airport before we even got on the plane. While in Vegas, I received an unexpected voicemail that my mom was getting remarried to a man I barely knew the following week. Another wave crashed.

Our bar crawl down the strip suddenly had a new level of motivation. Drown the sorrow. Drown the pain. Drown the dream of taking my future kids to the house I grew up in to see their grandparents for the holidays. Drown the identity crisis of feeling fractured because the ones who made me were broken apart.

When I try to describe depression to people, at least how it felt to me at this time, it was like my whole body was under water and my mouth was barely breaking the surface for air and I was struggling to stay afloat. It took immense amounts of effort to maintain the ability to breathe. If something dramatic or traumatic happened while already in this state, it was like a wave crashed over my already near drowning condition, causing me to sink lower and fight harder. The energy it took to simply stay in that breaking even state was almost too much.

It didn't feel like I had many healthy, secure attachments at the time to reach out to. I felt like I must internalize this struggle because I didn't want to bring anyone down with me. I decided to become the life of the party and was going to fake it till I made it through. As an adult with a decent income, I had easy access to self-destruction. I could afford the trouble I sought to get into. I even had a few companions who would find trouble with me. Even though the chronic insomnia had lifted, sleep was still a little evasive some nights, which meant weeknights were spent out a lot.

This out and about town lifestyle got expensive quick. Although I didn't want to (or honestly plan to at the time), I knew I needed to slow down, which again, had me motivated for my move to Nashville. I was going to let that mark the big change I needed. But until then, I was going to keep the party going.

My mom ended up marrying the stranger, whom we were all opposed to, a few short weeks after we found out his name. For some reason, this had a bigger wake than expected. I found myself going to church and then running to my car to let out a gut-wrenching cry for thirty minutes between service and singles Sunday school so I could possibly make it through the next hour. I couldn't balance it all anymore.

I reached out to one of my good friend's mothers, who was a family counselor and had always treated me like a daughter. She and her husband invited me to spend the next Sunday with them so I could get a break from everyone who knew me and just be. They sat on either side of me at their church and poured so much love into me. They fed me lunch and listened as I shared what was hurting. They prayed for me and helped me take a deep breath I had needed for a while.

Feeling this low and hopeless had taken a serious toll on how I felt about myself. I was disappointed in me. I thought, *I should be stronger than this. I'm an achiever. I'm a top performer. I am not supposed to be this weak.* They helped me see that I was human and not made to carry all I was trying to carry. They also reminded me I was never intended to go through this alone and that I wasn't. I hadn't put any trust in the One who was there because *I* was going to get myself through. *I* was always going to be there for myself. *I* didn't need anyone else. Such destructive independence. I see that now.

A BIG WEEK IN SEPTEMBER

Earlier in the year, it was announced that I earned top salesperson for my department nationwide, which came with a spectacular award of an all-expense paid vacation for me and a friend of my choosing. I invited Kim, one of my gal pals, and we planned to hit Mexico in style come September. I was so excited and told everyone who asked about my upcoming trip. Having something this big to look forward to also helped mask the deep depression lurking below the surface. In fact, if anyone were to ask how I was doing with any ounce of sincerity, I would have started crying.

Because of how emotionally fragile I was during this time, I tried to avoid any contact with mid-level acquaintances. I had my best friends close (who knew not to ask or at least when to ask) and then strangers. On September 2, 2002, I went to singles Sunday school with Kim and told her we couldn't sit by anyone I knew. I quickly scanned the room and saw a guy I didn't know, and it was as if he was under a spotlight. He looked like a visitor, so Kim and I went over to sit by him.

Thank God for shallow conversation at a round table. The guy's name was Ted, and he was, in fact, a visitor. As the Sunday school lesson went on, the teacher had questions for us to answer around the table. Great, I didn't have to talk about how I was doing. I asked Ted a few questions, to control the conversation, and found him to be noticeably honest. Something I found intriguing.

Of course, I told Ted about the upcoming trip we were set to depart for that week and get back Friday. We said our "so longs" and went our separate ways. Kim and I flew to Cabo the next day and checked out of reality for five unbelievable days. We flew back on Friday and both had the weekend off to recover from our vacation. The following Sunday, I told Kim we should look for that visitor again to sit by. As a card-carrying creature of habit, Ted was in the exact same seat.

I sat by him again and became more and more intrigued. Ted was so kind, honest, and humble, which wasn't the norm from my experience. He remembered I had my trip and asked how it went. That was even more impressive because it meant he actually listened when I told him the week prior. I didn't know all that was to come of this, but I knew I wanted to see him again. If these two weeks were any indication, he wouldn't be hard to locate.

9/11

On Tuesday morning, I woke up to a phone call from a friend telling me to turn on my television because a plane had crashed into one of the twin towers in New York City. I stared at the screen, watching smoke billow out when the second plane hit the second tower. There were no words to describe the disbelief, let alone the realization that this was no accident.

All major cities were told to evacuate key buildings and send people home. I worked in one of the more prominent buildings in Dallas, which was cleared just hours after I arrived for work. I returned to my apartment and spent the next eight or so hours alone watching the news, hoping it was all a bad dream. I couldn't feel anything.

For a normal person not dealing with undiagnosed depression, the events that transpired on September 11, 2001, brought grief, pain, fear, survivor's guilt, and many other normal feelings. For me, it gave a sense that nothing was sure in this life. Good people got up and went to work and never came home that day. I didn't want to be alone, but I also didn't want to crash in on any other family's time together while they mourned our country's loss. It amplified my current state a good bit. I went back and forth between comfort eating and no appetite, depending on the day.

The world outside of the cities directly affected by 9/11 slowly crept back to a new normal while everyone still carried the weight of trauma with them. The next several Sundays at church were expectedly somber. I didn't have to hold back any tears because many were crying. I wasn't the only one walking around virtually absent from the body anymore.

ONE LAST HOORAH

Due to the 9/11 attacks, the company I was working for no longer had plans to expand to Nashville that coming year. Everyone's growth plans were challenged as consumer spending shifted for a while. The job I was planning on moving with wasn't an option any longer, yet I knew I was still supposed to go. At this point, I was a mere three-and-a-half months away from Nashville, so I viewed my time left in Dallas as "for fun only."

In October, my three close friends took me out the night before my birthday for a one last hoorah dinner, which turned into a surprise party filled with a bunch of our small group and more. They made sure I didn't have an empty glass the whole night. By the time the party was supposed to move on to one of our favorite nightclubs, I was already drunk. Another of my friends worked the door at the club and made my designated driver take me home immediately. I was too drunk to enter. I told my friends (or at least I think I told them) to stay and have fun and I would go home.

I don't think I had been that drunk before. Between the lingering sadness of 9/11 and the nervousness about my move and leaving the life I knew, I didn't want to feel anything. My driver friend helped me into my apartment and brought me a glass of water and a trash can by my bed. I pulled off my fake eyelashes and fell asleep with plans of sleeping it off since the next day was Sunday.

8:00 a.m. the next morning, I woke up clear as a bell. How did that happen? Normally I, or anyone for that matter, would have been hurting from a serious hangover, but no. I felt oddly fantastic. I called a couple of my close friends to see if they were moving and no answer, so I went to church on my own. It was my birthday, and I wondered if Ted would remember since he remembered my trip to Mexico.

I walked into the Sunday school room, and the first person to greet me was Ted. He was waiting for me near the door. "Happy birthday," he said.

"Thank you! You remembered," I said.

I asked him if he wanted to sit by me since all my friends were recovering, and he said he wasn't staying for the class. His younger sister had her first baby, and he was going out to see them but came all the way to church just to tell me happy birthday. Wow! What? That was a long drive just for me.

He said, "I would have gotten you a gift, but my friends said that would look like I have the hots for you."

Without missing a beat, I asked, "And you don't?" totally sarcastically. Humor and sarcasm were my defaults.

His face turned all shades of red as he stuttered and tripped over his words. Equally embarrassed, I said, "I need to go to the bathroom," and ran off. I sat in the bathroom thinking: *Does he like me? Did I expose his feelings? I am moving to Nashville. This is horrible timing. Maybe I'll get a few free meals and some fun times before I tell him I'm moving.* I came back out of the bathroom, and we could hardly look at each other, yet, we were smiling from ear to ear. He wished me a happy birthday once again and then left to see his sister and new niece.

Two weeks later, I found myself in a similar situation where none of my usual friends made it to church due to a late and wild Saturday night. Thankfully, Ted was there, and we ended up sitting together again. It was becoming a regular thing. I asked him if he had any lunch plans after church, to which he awkwardly replied about promising his roommate he was going to fix a sink and maybe mow the lawn or something like that but had a conflicted look of wanting to see where my question was going.

I said, "Can you do that after lunch?"

He said, "I hadn't thought of that. Sure, I can do that stuff later."

We found a lunch place close by our church so we could take one car. Before getting out of the car, I felt compelled to tell him I was moving in now two months. In his words, I "shot his wheels off" because he was thinking we would get to know each other and become friends. Over that lunch, we proceeded to tell each other every crazy, awful, embarrassing thing we could think of about ourselves and our families. While Ted was talking, it felt like the restaurant got quiet, and I heard the words, "This is your husband." *What?! I don't even know him.* I paused Ted mid-sentence and asked, "Wait, what is your last name?"

He said, "Bradshaw," with a confused look on his face due to how random my question was.

In my head, I acknowledged what a great last name that was. *Charity Bradshaw,* I said to myself. I like the sound of that. Ted proceeded to share his story, and all I could think about was, *Am I the only one who knows? Does he know? This is only our first date; how can I even be thinking of marriage?* By Monday, we had plans for three dates that week. After all, I was moving soon. By Saturday, Ted knew I was the one for him, but we didn't talk about it because we didn't want to seem like psychopaths talking about marriage one week in.

Chapter Four

Everyone comes with baggage.
Find someone who loves you
enough to help you unpack.

UNKNOWN

Chapter Four
LOVE CHANGES EVERYTHING

This new love distracted me from all my sadness. I couldn't wait to see him and give him all my time and attention. Pretty soon, my usual gym time of two-hour workouts dwindled to only the days Ted was working because we were spending every waking, non-working moment together. I didn't realize how much new love could derail a fitness regimen, especially one that didn't have a good plan for the nutrition side of things. I was working out to negate a bad diet. At that age, it was somewhat doable, but wasn't a sustainable or long-term plan. It was like a hamster wheel I couldn't stop.

Between our eating out and ordering in, my weight started creeping back up. Ted, on the other hand, grew up skinny and had a fierce metabolism. In fact, his nickname was "Bones" in school. He pretty much burned through everything he ate even up to this point. There was something about this season of life where everything felt full of euphoric bliss. Food tastes better when enjoyed with someone you're falling for. I wanted him to experience my favorite Dallas spots before I left, and he was game for all of it.

Three weeks after our first date was Thanksgiving, on which Ted and I made plans to make the rounds and meet our respective families. He was going to cook the traditional meal for lunch at his place for his family, then we would have dinner at my mom's with her parents and my sisters, and then dessert with my dad, his partner, and his mom. The night before, we were chatting on the phone going over all the details when Ted made his intentions towards me very clear. He wanted me to be more than his girlfriend, and I wanted the same thing. So in a very informal yet meaningful way, we were engaged on November 22, 2001. A proper proposal, which caught me totally by surprise, came a little later.

Ted stayed up all evening cleaning his part of the house and preparing a meal for about fifteen people. It was nothing short of impressive, for me, romantic. His family was very welcoming, and lunch was a success. It wasn't until Ted's sister told him not to up and move to Nashville without saying something that he ever considered moving. He hadn't even thought of it yet, and I wasn't going to ask him to "move for me." I wanted it to be his idea—soon enough, it was.

We then made our way to my mom's house to eat again. I wasn't hungry, but that didn't matter. I didn't usually reserve the enjoyment of food for hunger alone. We typically did Mexican food for holidays because, well, it's awesome. When we arrived at her house, the first thing Ted saw was one of my sisters wracking my other sister's boyfriend. Literally, the first thing.

"Is she going to do that to me?" he asked with deep concern.

I said, "I hope not, but she might," and smiled to keep the suspense going.

More than anything, I wanted my grandparents' blessing that night. I wanted them to meet Ted and see if they saw what I saw in him despite not knowing him for very long. My grandma thought we should go around the table and all share what we were thankful for. With her brilliant strategic wit, she started with me so it would end with Ted. When it was Ted's turn, he stood up and said that first, he was thankful for his salvation and then ended with being thankful for me.

Without pause, my grandma exclaimed in front of everyone, "Yes, you can marry my granddaughter!"

We hadn't said anything to anyone, but my grandma knew. She even suggested we get married right away. Despite her highly persuasive methods and the fact that we had three ordained ministers in the house at that moment, we insisted on an actual wedding and having my grandparents officiate it. They agreed, and sooner than later, after coordinating all the schedules, we set a date—May 4, 2002.

Before Ted and I started dating, my free time was largely spent at the gym. After, most of my free time was spent with him, which wasn't great for my weight. By the time our wedding rolled around six months later, I was up about twenty-five pounds, yet Ted hadn't gained anything. Ted loved (and still loves) my curves, and I loved his svelte, lean body. We both got what we wanted in a spouse. In fact, besides his dreamy, oceanic aqua eyes, I saw Ted's great legs and immediately thought they needed to be duplicated.

I somehow had it in my mind that if I ate like Ted, a skinny person, I would be skinny too. There was plenty of confusing and misleading talk about how genetics don't play any role in metabolism, so I was convinced I could copy Ted in eating, and this would be my long-term weight management plan. Marrying a skinny person would solve my weight problems, and we would be an amazingly skinny and healthy couple together. It is easy to laugh at this thought now, but I truly believed it.

FOOD AND MONEY

Because 9/11 crushed my initial job plan in Nashville, I had to come up with another option. I didn't yet have a computer of my own, so I went to the library for hours a day looking for jobs and sending out resumes. For three months, I pounded the pavement, and nothing came in for me, so I took a job as a hostess at a restaurant near our apartment. I don't think I could have felt any lower. I was twenty-five years old with a college degree and national top salesperson status for my previous company, and at this point, I was working largely alongside teens not old enough to drive making $5.25 an hour.

My two-week paycheck wasn't enough to even pay for our groceries, so I started cleaning apartments in our complex and a house of a church friend. It was about this time I was approached to start a booking agency for upstart bands with some music businessmen. I saw potential in the idea, and rather than come in as an employee, I asked for partnership. This decision meant I would forgo a salary until the business was profitable as my sweat investment. I was now working full-time building a booking agency, making no money, part-time as a hostess, and then cleaning apartments and a house. Three jobs. I don't think I have ever worked so much.

Ted left a part-time pizza delivery job and came to Nashville with no degree or sales status and got a management job in three days. While I was thankful for his job and the income, it was a gut punch for my ego. Between my three jobs and Ted's job, we were still leaking financially. Every month we were out more than we were making and desperately needed to get things in order.

Before we married, we discussed everything including our finances. I had money in the bank, and Ted had around $40k in debt from what we called his "young and dumb" mistakes. His current spending behavior wasn't bad, but there were several things we needed to correct. He wanted to wait until he had the debt all paid off before we got married, and I didn't want to wait that long. I convinced him we could pay it off faster together. After a while, Ted came around and reluctantly agreed.

He didn't want me to feel the weight or burden of his debt, and I was sure it wasn't going to be a big deal. And it wasn't, until the debt collectors started calling a month after we were married. I quickly learned I was in over my head and out of my depth regarding how to get us out of this hole, so I asked a business friend if he had any suggestions on where we could go for help. He suggested we check out a financial class, so we did.

In July, only two months after our wedding, we joined. We barely had enough money to pay for the class, but we knew it was the right choice. We learned ways to reduce our bills and became aware of how much money we spent on things— including food. One of the mindsets I carried with me, even from childhood, was to not waste food. Somehow, I acquired scarcity thoughts subconsciously that contributed to not only me cleaning my plate but if there were free bread, chips, or whatever, I would eat my money's worth. The more I ate, the better the value, I believed.

For the sake of our budgeting purposes, the food we ended up "affording" ourselves was cheap and highly processed. Our special occasion eating out shifted to super-sized, fast-food meals. It didn't take long for me to not recognize myself. Of course, Ted's weight wasn't affected, and that wasn't fair. I was furious with him for having, in my mind, what seemed to be the ultimate male privilege of a faster metabolism.

WAKE-UP CALL

While I loved being in love, there were so many additional stressors that came with moving, marriage, debt, and money issues piling on top of the other issues I had but hadn't dealt with. Within less than a year, the toll of being on birth control, eating garbage, and the exhaustion from working three jobs added up to an additional fifty pounds. I remember getting into bed one night and looking down at my legs. They didn't even look like my legs. They were so swollen and puffy. Where had my muscles gone? I pushed on them with my pointer finger like they were dough while in sheer disbelief.

I cried out of shame, fear, and a heavy feeling of being so lost. Even though much of this change was good, I was having a hard time coping. I couldn't make it through a day without several unprovoked crying spells. If you'd have asked, I couldn't tell you why I was crying, and I certainly couldn't make myself stop.

It felt like my logical brain was talking to my emotional brain saying, "Pull yourself together. Don't be weak. You've got to stop crying. You are embarrassing me. This is not who we are." And my emotional brain was like a pile of goo on the floor, unable to move, unable to change, unable to regulate. Stuck.

I told Ted I was tired of crying every day. I didn't feel like my usual self, and I didn't know how to help myself. I went to a general practitioner and shared that I didn't know what was going on with me, and maybe I was sick or something. She handed me a questionnaire, and as I answered the questions, it was as if the person who wrote them knew exactly what was going on. My doctor tabulated the results, and it said I had severe depression. Depression? At the time, I thought that was for people who were weak-minded, as an excuse to get out of responsibility. That couldn't be me. I was duty-bound, dependable, and strong.

Depression wasn't exactly talked about or understood back then. I didn't know anyone else who ever had depression, so I had no grid for what it was like, how to get out of it, where it came from, etc. While it wasn't the answer I expected, I was glad to know it wasn't my imagination. I started a low-dose antidepressant and felt relief within days. I knew I didn't want to be on them permanently, but at least long enough to sort out my feelings while not while not having that drowning sensation.

Once I started feeling better emotionally, Ted and I began adding a few things to the calendar. Until then, I only had the mental space and energy for necessities. Our church had a worship night offered at the Ryman in downtown Nashville. I was excited to go, which was something I hadn't felt in a while. After it was over, it was chilly outside, so we did our best to hustle from the venue to the parking area. We were smiling and commiserating about the cold when all the sudden, I had to slow down. I couldn't keep up with the pace, and then I felt like I couldn't breathe.

It was a Sunday night, and nothing was open in the downtown area. We were still far from the car, and I was scared. Ted was trying to comfort and help me along, but I felt trapped. We needed to get to the car but walking up the incline to get there felt impossible. Not only was I in the middle of an asthma attack, but my total lack of strength wasn't helping. This was a newfound low. How did I get here? How did I get to where my clothes didn't fit and my knees and back hurt chronically? It felt like only a blink until the realization of how far I had let myself go sank in. I knew something had to change; I just had no idea how I to do it.

We decided to embark on a weight loss challenge together. Ted wanted to lose about ten to fifteen pounds, and I wanted to lose seventy. We watched a very inspirational advertisement video about an intense plan called *Body for Life*. It came with workouts and nutrition guides, and we were going to do this! If we wanted to, we could even compete in the plan's transformation contest. I have nothing negative to say about this program. It was helpful for people then and still helps people. It is extreme, and for some, this is exactly what they need.

After about a month on the program, Ted had surpassed his goal, and I was stuck at seven pounds down. He could eat nearly twice the amount I could, which made me furious (read jealous, and my inner child was pretty upset). He was melting, and I was frozen. I didn't have the mental stamina at the time to keep going on a program that felt like it was only working for one of us. One random Tuesday, a gal in my office decided she was going to join WeightWatchers® and attend a meeting during her lunch break, and somehow, I said I wanted to go too. I had heard a lot of good things about it and thought I could do it with her as my diet buddy.

In its purest form, there is so much good about WeightWatchers; however, for me, it became a game. I started looking for the "cheapest" foods that would satisfy my cravings for junk. Highly processed, low-fat, nutritionally vapid foods replaced the other junk I was eating. I lost around sixty pounds at the peak of my membership with them, which seemed like a success, but I wasn't learning to nourish myself; I was learning how to replace one junk food with another lower-calorie version. I do not fault WeightWatchers for my deficiency. I'm sure their materials had so much information about balanced meals and healthy eating, but I skipped that part because it sounded like punishment.

My inner child, who did most to all the driving in the food department, wasn't about to be put in the corner. She didn't go away despite the mild discipline I was operating in; she lurked around right below the surface, waiting for any moments of weakness. She knew our history and knew it was a matter of patience before she could get her way again.

KICKED OUT

I know, I know, you're wondering what it takes to get kicked out of WeightWatchers. For me, it took one simple and common thing for someone in my stage of life—pregnancy. Ted and I had been married a couple of years by this point and were finally on the same page regarding starting our family. We thought we would try for a while and eventually get pregnant. Surprise! The first month we tried, we succeeded. I was so excited to share this with my WeightWatchers family but was not prepared for the news that I would have to leave the program. They said I could come back once the baby was born, and I could do the nursing mothers version, but that left me out on my own again for months.

While I could rationalize the legal aspect of their demand, I was in a slight tailspin. I had been in this program for around a year at this point. I had my community taken away from me when I needed them the most. I did not do well on my own, so this felt personal. My inner child was getting the food party ready for us, but sadly, it was delayed a few months due to morning sickness. Once month four hit, my appetite was back, and I was feeling good. The whole pregnancy metabolism thing was awesome. At my OB visit, I saw I didn't gain any weight for my first trimester, which the inner child took as a license to EAT! I thought, since I can't diet right now, I can eat whatever I want because being pregnant would burn it off.

Operation "eat the stuff I haven't eaten for the last year" was in full swing. I felt invincible. At my next OB appointment, four weeks later, the scale said I had gained seven pounds. I rationalized that as I didn't gain ANY weight for three months so in fact this is like gaining seven pounds in four months. That's pretty good, I thought to myself. The next OB appointment, also four weeks later, another seven pounds appeared. Then another, and another, and another.

By the time I was full term, I had gained forty pounds. This didn't truly scare me because I naively thought I would have an eight-pound baby, plus a few pounds for the placenta, and would be halfway down before even leaving the hospital. Then with breastfeeding, the rest would melt off in a month or two—nothing to worry about here. I even told friends I planned to be my pre-pregnancy weight within three months. Their faces told a story that I didn't want to read.

Our birth plan was for everything to be as natural as possible. I had a doula, and all my sisters and mother were in town since our son was the first grandchild born on our side of the family. At forty weeks, he showed no signs of wanting to be born, so my doctor began discussions of inducing labor and what that would look like. At forty-one weeks, my doctor wasn't comfortable waiting any longer, so she scheduled us to come in that night for an induction. We were nervous and excited. I was ready to be delivered but also terrified of the exit options.

Being induced overnight meant I didn't sleep at all. Between the nerves and the blood pressure cuff going off every fifteen minutes, there was no rest or relaxation to be had. The induction medication required constant monitoring, which I wasn't fully aware of when I agreed to it. This meant going into the day our first child was to be born completely exhausted.

At 5:30 a.m. the following morning, the nurses began running Pitocin, which created contractions since my body wasn't in labor. I declined pain medication because I wanted this to be a "natural" birth, not realizing it was very medical already. After twelve-plus hours of mind-blowing pain, the doctor let us know our son wasn't tolerating the path we were on and began prepping me for an emergency c-section. Physically exhausted, I demanded that I not feel another contraction and told them to give me whatever I needed for surgery immediately. I couldn't take the suffering of another one. I and my plan had failed.

With the epidural in place, they wheeled me into the operating room where I fell in and out of sleep. Ted was brought in once they were ready to begin. About three minutes later, our son was born healthy and whole, but I missed nearly all of it. I couldn't keep my eyes open from being so tired and medicated. All I could think of was I didn't do the one thing I set out to do, which was be able to have my baby with my mom and sisters in the room with me. I let them down. I let myself down. I felt I let everyone down. *My mom had all four of us naturally, why couldn't I do it? It must be because I wasn't woman enough, strong enough, whatever enough.*

Rather than leaving the hospital with that can-do I thought I would have, I left exhausted, recovering from being cut open, ashamed, and alone. Our family had to leave the day after he was born because of going so long overdue. My unrealistic expectations were crushing me. I set myself up with such high hopes that there was nowhere to go but failure. This didn't bode well for my weight. We had virtually no support system at the time, outside of one friend, who would pick up whatever we wanted from Sonic° on her way home from work to help take care of us.

While I did deliver an eight-pound baby, the scale didn't care. Those forty pounds quickly became fifty, then fifty-five. I was running my struggling small business at the time, which meant no paid maternity leave. Everything felt hard, so eating became the comforter. Those pounds had nowhere to go. I continued wearing maternity clothes for a while and then eventually acquiesced to buying larger sizes—again.

THE POUNDS KEPT STACKING UP

We were genuinely enjoying being parents. Our son figured out sleeping through the night quickly and had a general ease to him. We thought we were experts right out of the gate. Mildly terrified of getting pregnant again so easily, I tried to go on the pill again, and it made me feel crazy and gain weight. I quickly came off it, and we decided to do natural family planning for a while. While we didn't want to get pregnant right away, as we were enjoying life with one, we eventually wanted to grow our family. When our son was about one year old, we decided to start casually trying again for number two.

During this time, I left the music industry and sent my small business out to pasture. After searching for what my next stage would be, I decided to go to cosmetology school. I still wanted to work for myself; I wanted something a little more personal and creative. By now, our casual trying turned a little more serious as we weren't getting pregnant. Several months into serious trying, we came up short with no pregnancy. I automatically assumed it was my fault. My physical condition was hindering us from this next baby. I found myself slipping back into the darkness once again.

Month six—no baby. Month eight—no baby. Month ten—no baby. Finally, I did the only thing I knew to do at that time— go back to WeightWatchers. I began losing weight again and started feeling a little better about myself. We stopped trying and gave the unromantic "duties" a break. I celebrated the first fifteen pounds down and was about to buy a three-month pass for WeightWatcher meetings when low and behold, thirteen months later, I found out I was pregnant. Guess who got kicked out again.

I did my best to "do better" this pregnancy. I had a similar first trimester but tried to avoid some of the gaining I did with the first pregnancy. I didn't know what kind of exercise I could do safely other than walking or elliptical, so I ended up focusing on those. I did about forty minutes of cardio several times a week until a month out. I knew I would have to take some time off from doing hair after delivery, so I worked as much as possible right up until days before I had her.

Between the exercise and my busy work schedule, I gained only twenty-five pounds this time and had a nearly ten-pound baby via c-section again due to the risks with her size. She ate and slept like a champ from the beginning because she was a bigger baby, which made some things easier from the start. I was excited to start losing again, but despite all these weight loss meetings, I never actually addressed the root of my problem, so my problem was there waiting for me.

After baby number two, I only lost the actual baby weight. The other fifteen remained. I was exhausted, which I didn't have an explanation for since she was sleeping so well, and I was getting way more rest than with our son. Several months went by before I finally went and had some blood work done to see if there were any underlying issues. My doctor referred me to an endocrinologist who explained I might have had a thyroid condition called Hashimoto's thyroiditis. It is an autoimmune condition where the body attacks its own thyroid causing it to not produce enough thyroid hormones, which lead to fatigue, weight gain, hair loss, and many other symptoms.

I thought, *THIS IS WHY! This is why I "can't" lose weight. This is my problem* (my excuse, actually). I was sure the doctor was going to give me medication to fix everything and make me skinny like I was supposed to be. Sadly, to me, she didn't put me on medication right away. I was bummed. She wanted to watch my levels as she said it could have been exacerbated by pregnancy. I did blood work two more times over the next few months, and for the final one, the letter I received said my blood work looked normal and no medication was needed.

Dang it. I wanted skinny pills. But oh well. I felt better and that was something. One Saturday morning, our son was pushing four years old, our daughter was nine months old, and I was feeling tired again. This didn't make sense since I had recently received that letter saying my thyroid was normal. *Wait. No way. Do I have any tests here at the house?* My brain was reeling at the possibility. Between my thyroid being off, still breastfeeding, and watching the calendar, we thought our chances of getting pregnant were slim to none. Yet, sure enough, I found out I was ALREADY pregnant, and our new daughter was only nine months old!

Oh, my Lord! Our daughter wasn't even walking yet. We weren't mad about being pregnant, just totally caught off guard. I couldn't even think about losing weight at this point. I focused on trying to not gain any during this pregnancy. My weight was at a cumulative high, and my doctor told me I didn't need to gain any weight to support a healthy pregnancy. I tried my best to follow her advice and only gained fifteen with my third pregnancy.

Our newest daughter was born healthy and at a normal weight. For some reason, I worried about her because I was pregnant so soon after my second baby. I didn't know if there were enough nutrients left or if she would get less than optimal stuff from me since I was still recovering and rebalancing. There I was with a four-year-old, a seventeen-month-old, and a newborn. Tired didn't even begin to describe how I was feeling. I knew I wanted to feel better and have more energy as the demands of motherhood were steep at the time, but I had no idea where to start. It was like I was floating or drifting away with nothing to anchor to.

A dear friend, who was a personal trainer, saw the tailspin I was in and offered to train me. I was so excited. I looked forward to every session because she was so positive, and I didn't have to do it alone. When we couldn't meet in person, she would email me what to do, and I would always follow her instructions. It was like I could do whatever someone else told me to do but couldn't come up with it on my own. Foodwise, I was still looking at how to cheat the system and get as many food rewards as I could possibly find. Calories burned were calories earned, and I could justify eating them. While I wasn't doing as much as I could have correctly, I still managed to lose nearly forty pounds, which was about what I gained from the last two pregnancies.

Chapter Five

If you don't make time for your wellness, you'll be forced to make time for your illness.

UNKNOWN

Chapter Five
THE DARK AGES

Despite being down forty pounds and much more active, tiredness crept back in. Back to the endocrinologist I went. The same thing was determined with pregnancy related thyroid issues that resolved after several more months. In August of that year, our children were five years, two years, and eight months old. My husband, after much prayer and deliberation, entered nursing school, and I became the breadwinner and now homeschool mom of our oldest. One of the biggest reasons we homeschooled at first was because the thought of waking up early every day to put him on the bus truly felt insurmountable. I needed every minute of sleep at this point in my life, so homeschooling him meant later mornings and a more casual schedule.

This stage of life was very dark for me. Ted was covered up with reading and studying because the nursing programs were so rigorous. He felt so much internal pressure to get As and didn't want to fail our family. I was working, homeschooling, and hauling three kids to nearly everything alone. The grocery store was a nightmare; I had nowhere to put all the food we needed, plus the baby carrier, and trying to wrangle the older two. I tried two carts one time and ended up crying at the register. I had no social life. It felt too awkward to hang out with married friends as the only one from our couple, not to mention with the three young kids in tow.

I was sad. The kind of sad that doesn't see a way out. Nursing school was a long-term commitment of over four years, and we were only in year one. The days were long, very long. Every area of my life was stretched to nearly the breaking point. Yet food was always there for me. It was there when I was lonely. It was there when I was sad. It was there when I was stressed and there when I was mad. It didn't judge me or ask me for a reason or excuse. It could be whatever I needed it to be.

"PERFECT" TIMING

After a couple of years, the burden of Ted's school demands became more bearable. I don't know if I got stronger or the children growing up some played into it, but alas, I was happy for somewhat easier. Ted had several semesters under his belt and many of the difficult classes behind him. We found ourselves with enough time and energy to get pregnant yet again. Our youngest was two at the time, so this was a perfect age difference. I excitedly told my family and was wonderfully surprised to find out I was pregnant at the same time as my sister. Our due dates were nearly the exact same. This was especially fun since our last children were only three days apart as well.

Since this was my fourth pregnancy, my doctor didn't need to see me until I was about ten weeks along. I hadn't had any issues with my prior pregnancies, so no rush. We were heading into winter, and I was especially cold, which wasn't my norm when a bun was in my oven. Ted chalked it up to the weather, but something in me didn't see it that way. The wait to ten weeks felt especially long because of this concern. I simply wanted confirmation that everything was okay.

The day of our "first peek" appointment finally came around, and it began with an ultrasound. Having seen plenty of these before, I could immediately tell something wasn't right. The baby did have a heartbeat, but it was smaller than I thought it would be by ten weeks. We were sent over to our doctor's office where she shuffled through her due date calculator and asked me more questions. While she didn't seem distressed, she did look puzzled. She set our next appointment for a few weeks after the holidays, when we would return from traveling. A short time, which felt like an extremely long wait.

I still had my concerns and suspicions, but Ted wasn't worried. He said he wasn't going to worry until they gave him a reason to. While we were traveling, Ted and our brothers-in-law went to a professional basketball game with our son. I was tired due to being toward the end of my first trimester, so I went to bed. While lying there relaxing, my heart started beating rapidly. I didn't know what was happening, but it felt like I was running a race yet not moving. After about an hour, it eventually subsided, and I fell asleep. There were no other issues in the gap between appointments.

We returned to our doctor only to be escorted to the "other" hallway. This wasn't the "happy" hallway. It was off to the other side of the waiting room, so it would be less visible. The attendant walked us back for our ultrasound. I noticed on my paperwork the word "viability" but didn't think anything of it at the time. Minutes later, we were looking at the screen, seeing the same-sized baby, but now there was no heartbeat. The baby stopped growing on the exact day of our last ultrasound. I started crying while Ted could only stare at the screen in disbelief. He looked like he was trying to make medical sense of what was happening, but there wasn't any to be found. We had miscarried.

This wasn't what I had in mind for my perfect plan, to be done having children by thirty-five when all the risks are lowest. That plan was now impossible. Having another "twin cousin" with my sister was impossible. Having a perfect pregnancy record was impossible. This hit hard. I couldn't be happy for any of my friends who were pregnant at the time. I didn't want to go anywhere. *How could I be singled out like this? Why even let me get pregnant at all if it was going to end this way?* I was mad at God, the world, and everything happy. I had about fifteen pounds of pregnancy weight but no baby to show for it. Sadness eating was almost my sport at this point.

I wasn't sure if we were going to try again. I had always wanted four children, not exactly sure why. While I was hurting and mourning our loss, I didn't feel our story would end this way. We followed the doctor's advice and gave my body the time needed to heal and recover. I did need something to look forward to, though, so we decided I would plan our first real trip as a married couple for our tenth anniversary. Can you say all-inclusive in Riviera Maya? We had been working so hard for so long between school, my business, kids, and now add a miscarriage; this break was truly what we needed. Because we were watching my cycles, I noticed this trip spanned my ovulation window. I told Ted so he could mentally prepare, as I didn't want to get pregnant and not be able to enjoy a drink here or there on our trip.

A RAINBOW

We arrived at our resort, and I immediately felt the stress melt off. We made time to laugh, compete in resort games, rest, but also to cry as we were finally able to be alone and process everything. Apparently, we had such a good time that we brought home a little souvenir, our tenth anniversary special. We were pregnant. I was reluctant to tell anyone as the news of a miscarriage was hard to share. It did seem that as soon as I peed on the stick, my stomach already looked pregnant, which was unfair. I wanted to keep it a secret for a few months. I soon started getting the "You're glowing," comments and looks of "Are you going to tell us something?" All I knew was this was going to be my last pregnancy, and I was determined to enjoy it.

I switched OBs for this one because of how things ended in the negligent care of our miscarriage. Our new doctor was absolutely outstanding. He was the best. From our first appointment, he prayed for us, our baby, and the entire pregnancy. I didn't know he was a Christian when I switched over, but it was a wonderful addition to all his already stellar qualities. We shared what happened with our last pregnancy, and he promised me he would do whatever it took for me to have a stress-free experience this go around. I held him to it.

My sister had her baby when I was about three months along. I planned a trip out to meet her newborn son but had to get some information first. If this last pregnancy was a girl, I was going to take all my baby boy clothes out to her as I wouldn't need them anymore. I begged my doctor to give me my ultrasound earlier than twenty weeks so I could know if I was taking all this stuff or not. He let me have my scan at eighteen weeks, a day before my trip out.

We brought our three kids to the appointment so we could find out what it was together. After about ten seconds, I could see we were having a girl, but I also noticed they were spending a lot of time looking at her brain, spine, hands, and umbilical cord. *What was the concern? What did they see?* I asked the ultrasound tech, but she wasn't allowed to answer. She simply said we would need to wait for the geneticist to come in and discuss it with us. *Geneticist? Why not the regular ultrasound reader?* Because our kids were present, I felt the need to hold back the tears so as not to scare them. I turned to Ted and paused as we both exchanged concerned looks. I went to the bathroom attached to our patient room and silently wept for the few minutes I had before pulling it back together.

The geneticist came in and consulted with us on our baby's condition. She had a couple areas of concern like cysts on her brain and a single vessel umbilical cord. Individually, these things aren't so bad, but together, they had concerns for genetic abnormalities. They said she looked good otherwise, but we would need to monitor her growth due to the single vessel cord and wait to see if the cysts resolve on their own, which could happen. I went into this ultrasound thinking all we would discover would be whether our baby was a boy or girl, not that there were heavy issues. It took my breath away a bit, but I had to keep going so I could pack up all our boy clothes and get ready to meet my new nephew.

I flew out to Phoenix by myself, which gave me a slight break from my day-to-day routine and busyness. Every time I got preoccupied with concern over my pregnancy and our baby's health, my sister would bring my nephew over for me to hold. It was sort of a reset and refocus on something joyful and precious. He was a wonderful distraction.

I don't know when I officially decided, but at some point, I determined to enjoy this pregnancy and did my part as much as I could. It was different being older with this pregnancy. All my paperwork said "advanced maternal age" as if suddenly I were an old woman doing a young woman's activity. I told my doctor my history of pregnancy weight gain and concern, and he was very gracious through the whole process. While I did end up gaining thirty pounds with this baby, I tried to focus on not worrying and remaining positive.

At a late ultrasound, we saw that the cysts had resolved, and her growth was perfectly normal. She looked perfect. Her c-section was the smoothest and happiest as my doctor sang

"Happy Birthday" to her as she was born. I was able to nurse her immediately after I was finished in the operating room, and the biggest wave of relief covered me. I am thankful I had faith that things would be alright. That was against my usual nature at the time. Worrying came easier, but I knew that wouldn't help my baby. Knowing she would be our last, I cherished everything about it from nursing to diapers, spit-up to outfit changes. She had two sisters who barely let a peep out of her because they would race to her side and see what she needed. It was a very sweet and endearing season.

BODY ISSUES

One thing different about this c-section and this doctor was that he sent me home with my staples in place rather than removing them before I went home. This wasn't a big deal until I had to take my first shower and caught a glimpse of what I looked like. The postpartum belly, for someone who was already overweight, was nothing I ever enjoyed seeing. But add what looked like a metal braces smile to it and it brought me to ugly tears. I had to hold my skin up to see the staples, which made me cry. It looked like the smile was laughing because of the way my stomach moved when I cried, which made me cry even more. By this time, I had almost forgotten that I came into the bathroom to shower. Before going into the bathroom, I'm sure I had some idea that my stomach looked like a trainwreck, but I didn't have any idea of how I actually looked. It was as if a tire had gone flat like a doughnut on my belly.

After the initial shock had worn off and the staples were removed, I settled into my "new look" of deflated belly and kind of made peace with it. In a strange way, I had sort of a reverse body dysmorphia. I didn't think I was "that bad." While ignorance may have been bliss, my physical condition had consequences. One of the big complications I had to deal with was sagging skin and the side effects that came with it. I didn't know it at the time, but I had a skin condition that caused painful lesions, and they were exacerbated by overlapping skin or areas where bacteria could easily grow. I got repeated infections in my c-section scar area due to this condition and the amount of hanging skin I had. This meant antibiotics, powders, and special medical fabric to put between the folds of skin to keep it dry.

Let me tell you what this regimen did for my self-esteem. There is nothing more humbling than powdering between the skin folds, then putting a medical-grade fabric in place, just so you won't get an infection living your normal life that day. I couldn't even talk about it because I was so embarrassed. I would try to be sure Ted wasn't around when it came time to doctor up my underbelly. What for some might be considered a vanity issue was covered in medical complications that became annoying and exhausting.

Another issue I dealt with during this time was a ton of back pain. I could no longer sit or lay down without pain. The only thing that didn't hurt was standing, but I couldn't stand all the time. I couldn't sit down during church, mealtime, or while driving without significant pain. Sometimes I didn't know if I could stand up after sitting for a while because of the pain I had to push through. I had a physiotherapist friend who would work on me as she could, but it would only do so much. This pain was from a few bulging discs and both S.I. joints in my lower back being inflamed and angry. This kind of pain will make you try anything and everything to get out of it, from steroid packs to ultrasound-guided injections, but nothing was working long-term.

I met with a non-surgical orthopedist who diagnosed me with diastasis recti, which is basically a separated abdominal wall down the middle. He prescribed more physiotherapy and a prescription anti-inflammatory but was certain surgery would be the only thing that could correct it. Since I was very afraid of surgery in general, I decided to do all the other things I could to address the issue and see if that would work at resolving the near unbearable pain. I thought the cause of my back pain was relegated to a structural problem. I didn't quite yet link my weight as a contributor, much less a large contributor to it. With the diastasis diagnosis, I thought it was an abdominal wall support issue and that was it.

CONSIDERING ALL MY OPTIONS

Nothing was working. I had done everything I was told to do, but nothing moved the needle on the pain scale. One of my clients worked for a plastic surgeon who was one of the best in Nashville. During her appointment with me, she mentioned him when I brought up my struggle and diagnosis. She suggested I at least talk with him and see what he advised. She said he was very conservative and honest and not desperate to add patients to the calendar. That made me feel at ease, so I scheduled a consultation.

Not going to lie, I thought if I was brave enough to have the surgery, he could take all this belly skin off me, cinch up my abdominal wall, and it would be like I never had kids or a pooch. I started romancing the idea and getting mildly excited about it. I pushed the stroller with my then six-month-old baby into the doctor's office after filling out paperwork and waiting a few minutes for the doctor. By this point, surgery with this doctor had become my solution. I was ready to say yes to fixing this mess, but I was trying to play it cool and not seem too eager.

He walked in and was very nice and professional. I told him my situation, and he agreed surgery was likely the option that would fix the diastasis issue. It felt like everything was going in the right direction until I asked him if I was a good candidate for this, and he said, "No." Suddenly my fantasy of not having a blob of goo in my midsection or the terrible back pain from it was ripped from my hands with that single word. It was like I was dancing at a party, and someone pulled the plug on the music. He continued the consultation by explaining I had too much visceral fat (fat around my organs) and that I needed to lose at least forty pounds, but more would be better. He suggested I lose all the weight I would want to lose in that range and then return for another consultation.

He also casually noted my weight was likely aggravating my back and was part of the problem. While I know that might have been challenging for someone to say to a stranger, I could tell he cared and wanted me out of pain, so I appreciated the risk he took. This information completely shifted my focus to "I must lose weight so I can have this surgery." I wanted to get there as soon as possible, so my next consideration was weight loss surgery (WLS). I didn't feel like I could "control" my eating habits anyway, so I could have surgery, and it would force me to eat smaller meals! Since I had already gotten myself psyched to have one surgery, what's another?

I found a bariatric practice in Nashville and scheduled Ted and me to attend the required meetings before scheduling surgery. The first presentation went through the four or so variations of WLS, which was a little gruesome to me. It was like wanting to eat a bacon burger but then finding out exactly how they are made, causing you to lose your appetite. I barely made it out upright of the presentation but was able to check it off the list of requirements. I then scheduled the one-on-one consultation and was told I was not "unhealthy enough" to be a candidate. If I were ten to fifteen pounds heavier or had comorbidities, I would be a candidate to have it covered by insurance.

All I wanted was help, and it felt like no one would help me. *Should I try to gain weight to get the surgery? Is that insane to even think?* Also, the information about permanent malnutrition, vomiting, diarrhea, and more on the other side of WLS scared me. *What if, at some point, I didn't have access to the vitamins and supplements needed to maintain organ function?* The surgery itself had a one percent mortality rate at the time, which meant one person in every one hundred died, either on the table or as a result of complications after. That hit too close for me. I had four kids and a husband; I didn't want to die, so I dismissed the idea of WLS—at least for a little bit.

I had piles of intention and knew I was going to change. I had to. I had eaten poorly for so long that it got me to this place of pain and shame. I can now look back and have grace for who I was then. I was homeschooling two kids with a third, who was especially curious and wanted to learn, along with an infant, while working full time and putting my husband through nursing school. It. Was. Crazy. Every candle was burning at every end. I ended up choosing meals I knew the kids wouldn't balk at, which often meant they were not in the direction of my goals. I chose the path of least resistance when resistance was what would have started adding up. I didn't have the energy to fight the kids to eat or me to eat better. The inner child was well-fed and fully armed with reasons these were the right choices. I was tired.

Chapter Six

Your past is not your
present or your potential.

ELIZABETH BENTON

Chapter Six
A FRESH START

COLD TURKEY

Thankfully, Ted's time in school was ending. We were excited to be nearing the dual-income phase again, and right in time because we needed a larger house. We had gone from three of us when we bought it to now seven while Ted's dad lived with us. I looked and looked but couldn't find a house that had what we needed for a price we could swing at the time. It was very frustrating. I felt trapped, and no one likes that feeling.

In the middle of all this, Ted and I were invited to come and speak at a relationships conference in Houston where my mom and sister lived. We were honored and excited for the opportunity to do something like this together. We were encouraged to write a book about marriage through this event and released *Staying I Do* a few years later.

While we both were very happy with our careers, we always looked for ways to work together. During our time there, we felt like we were supposed to sow financially into the ministry hosting us as a seed for direction about a house, and that direction came faster than we imagined. Two days later, we were back in Nashville grabbing something we needed for the house. As we were walking to our car, I asked Ted how he felt while we were in Texas. He kind of shrugged and said he felt fine. I told him I felt like we were supposed to move to Houston (which was on our "never do" list, so watch out when you say never). He quickly agreed.

Did that just happen? A five-minute conversation turned into a cross-country move. This didn't make any sense but gave us both so much peace. This conversation happened in mid-August of 2014. Ted had four months until he graduated, which gave us four months to get everything buttoned up. We put our house on the market ourselves and sold it to the first couple who viewed it the week of Thanksgiving! If you know anything about real estate, you know what a big deal that was. It was happening. We were moving. This was a perfect chance for me to "start over."

I made up my mind, when we moved to Texas, I would never eat bad food again. That's how I was going to change my life. It made so much sense—new place, new habits, new life. Never mind that with me, as always, was me. It wasn't Nashville making me eat poorly. I'm sharing this in case you have ever made an impossible promise to yourself but didn't have to publicly acknowledge it. You're not alone.

We held graduation parties and attended going away parties along with holiday parties, and I am not sure I even weighed myself for a solid month. I might have even packed the scale early to get ahead of the game. I was living life with no limits because after the move, the party was over.

One important thing to note was I couldn't bring my business with me (as much as I would have loved to import many of my clients). I was committing to a fresh business start as well. I was going from breadwinner to I'm not sure in minutes. My plan was to "burn my ship" of sorts and sell nearly all my hair gear, outside of what it would take to keep up my family. I would no longer be identified or branded a hairstylist. Some other career was coming my way.

One of the biggest reasons I wasn't going to do hair full-time anymore was due to the pain and inflammation I had in my hands, wrists, and shoulders. I couldn't see a way to scale myself in hair, and I knew I wanted to have a greater impact than that as well as a new creative outlet. I had been doing hair for nearly a decade, and my body needed a break on so many levels.

WHERE TO LAND?

We didn't want to buy a house right away because we weren't sure what area of Houston we wanted to land in, so we moved into my mom's house for what we thought would be a couple of months. We searched for a house, and nothing surfaced that met our needs. We even adjusted a few and still nothing. We also had to face financing issues since our financial situation changed so much, and Ted had to wait for a hospital job to come along. This took a little longer than usual since he was brand new with no experience and no local relationships as he had in Nashville from his clinical rotations.

Nothing was panning out the way we thought it would. One thing we did decide on was to put our school-aged kids into public school to help them make friends. They were starting over too, and we wanted them to integrate and meet friends as soon as possible. With the house hunting going flat, I told Ted if we could not find a place by the time school started, we would enroll them in my mom's district and wait the year out at her house. It wasn't too bad since she traveled much of the time. But it still was hard being a thirty-something couple with four kids living at a place that wasn't ours.

I was supposed to make my big change of no bad foods but was constantly surrounded by incoming treats, sweets, and more. My mom knew what our favorites were and kept them coming. It was like kryptonite. I felt all willpower leave my body.

A voice was rolling around in my head saying things like, *"You failed again. You made yourself a promise and didn't keep it. You can't trust yourself."*

These messages rang loud and clear along with many more. I beat myself up brutally.

"You deserve to be in pain. You deserve to feel ashamed. You don't deserve happiness, that's for sure. You're unlovable. You're hopeless. You're not worth the effort. You're disgusting."

Between the stress of all these things and my horrible self-talk, gaining another ten pounds was easy-peasy. With my income pretty much gone, no friends, no home of my own, no friends for my kids, and a few second thoughts, I felt worthless. It was another dark time. To make matters worse, within the first few months of us being there, our youngest broke her leg in an accident, our minivan door stopped working and needed almost $2k in repairs, and our son's front two permanent teeth got broke on a gym floor during a holiday when no offices were open. It literally felt like hell had broken loose—stress, stress, stress. My body didn't tolerate this well at all.

I decided, since I was up that extra ten pounds needed to be eligible for WLS, I would try to get up the nerve again and have one of the surgeries. Again, I attended the first required presentation, which was done in a large group style, and one of the points the presenter made hit me differently than the first presentation I attended. She said that after surgery, we still must learn to eat healthier meals and smaller portions and get our bodies moving to experience long-term success. That sounded a lot like what you would need to do *without* surgery. *Then why have the surgery? If I would still need to do what to me was the "hard work" of it, why take all that risk?*

(I will insert here that several of my friends and family members have had some variation of WLS, and some have successfully kept the weight off and have lived much improved lives because of it. Some have not. I am simply sharing my experience and thought process here. No judgment on those who have taken this route at all.)

I was relieved and sad that I no longer felt like WLS was an option for me. While I didn't want to undergo all the cutting, risk, and recovery, I did like the idea of weight melting off quickly and easily. To let go of that had a slightly low feeling to it. Ted and I walked out of the office together quietly. I am thankful for his consistent support through every consideration of my journey. He never pressured me to be anything other than me and accepted me at every stage. While sometimes this was a lot of room to roam around in, I do appreciate always feeling loved and worthy.

I wasn't feeling super awesome once again, so I decided to get some blood work done through my sister who is a naturopathic doctor (ND). My labs showed I did need to be on a thyroid prescription at this point as my body wasn't bouncing back like it had the other times, and my A1C was elevated into the pre-diabetic zone. A1C is a test that measures the average amount of sugar in your blood over the last three months and is used to help diagnose prediabetes and diabetes.[4] It was decided I would do best on medication to lower that into a healthier range as well. While I was glad to have some explanation of why I wasn't feeling great and some awareness of things I *could* be doing differently, I didn't change anything about how I was eating or moving. It was the typical "throw a pill at it" management solution.

THE "NEW HOUSE" PROMISE

Summer was coming to an end, and we still had no house prospects in sight as well as no grid for what we could afford at the time. My income went to virtually nothing, and Ted was at starter night nurse pay. While we didn't want it to be the case, it looked like we were going to be staying at my mom's for a while longer because school was starting soon. We enrolled the older three in fifth, second, and kindergarten, while the youngest stayed home with me. This was a huge adjustment for all of us. Ted was flipping back and forth between being asleep and awake during the day, the school kids were getting used to a new school and how a school works, and our youngest was adjusting to being the only kid at home with no one to play with.

I was adjusting to all of it. It was all new. Our youngest needed a lot of attention now that her three playmates were gone all day. Sometimes I felt like a single mom because Ted's sleeping schedule was all over the place, and his shifts varied weekly, putting me in charge of all things household and children. I was also finding my way into a new career. My mom had encouraged me to write a book for a while, and since I was no longer doing hair full-time, this was the opportunity to get that done. I ended up publishing three books that year, and in that process, I discovered I could help others write their books. I stumbled upon a niche that suited my skills and passion for helping people find their voice and the deep satisfaction of writing their stories. Finally, some light was shed on what seemed to be a very dark and difficult season.

Soon, what was all new became routine. It felt like we were in a groove and had some hope. In March 2016, we found a house in the area we wanted to land, and it met our wish list. We moved after school ended so the kids could finish the school year where they were. It was so exciting knowing we would once again have our own place where we could control what came in the house (re. food) and for it to be ours. While we are forever grateful for my mom's hospitality and generosity during this time, it was still hard for all of us. This new house was going to be a for-real life change. I wasn't going to buy any junk food. "No junk food in the new house" would be posted in all high-traffic areas. We would exercise every day. We would be the healthy people this time—I promise.

Moving day came, and we cleared out our storage unit along with our stuff at mom's house. A large group of our friends came and helped us with every part, from washing dishes and sheets to assembling bunk beds. Several even made lunch for all the helpers and our family. It was almost overwhelming how much generosity we received. We were used to being the ones helping. To be on the receiving end of things was quite different. In our usual fashion, we had the house unpacked in about three days and prepared for a party to ensure everything got put away quickly.

Little by little, the junk food crept in. It was maybe a "clean" food house for about three days. Another promise made to myself broken and thus reinforcing the bedrock belief that I couldn't trust myself. *Why did I even think I was serious? Who was I kidding? It's who I am and will always be.* Time to melt the queso and drown my shame in it.

ROCK BOTTOM

By the next fall, the kids had all started in their new schools including our youngest who went to a sweet Mother's Day Out program close by. This meant I had some time to get things done and not have to answer the thousands of questions kids can come up with so easily. In the stillness, I began noticing how I felt. I had no energy. Zero. There were days I could barely lift my arms much less get out of bed. It felt like death. *Am I depressed?* I didn't think so. Things were going great at the time. I didn't feel sad or overwhelmed like the previous seasons. This was so heavy and very concerning. I shared what I was experiencing with Ted and had him watch me for signs or symptoms of depression. We also decided it was probably a good idea to get bloodwork done again to see if there was anything physiological going on.

Low and behold, my iron level was dangerously low. This is common in people with thyroid issues, but when combined with torrential menstruation, it's no wonder I felt the way I did. My body couldn't keep up. Again, I was so excited to find out this was a physiological issue rather than psychological. I only needed more iron. I began taking a viable supplement, and while it helped some, it didn't fully catch me up to normal or optimal levels.

I had some options though. I could go regularly for iron infusions, or I could address the biggest culprit—my uterus. After months of deliberation and fighting the fear of "going under," I decided to see an OBGYN and have a consultation for a uterine ablation, which would likely remedy the iron issue in less than an hour. We knew we were done having children, so I didn't need to continue with these unbearable periods every month. I could keep all my parts while reducing the amount of blood by ninety to ninety-five percent each month. I was giddy thinking about not losing any day's activities to my period anymore. Everything could be yes after this. *Can I swim whenever I want? Yes! Can I sit on a cloth couch any day of the month? Yes!*

When I arrived at the appointment, the first thing they did, per usual, was check my weight. I hadn't been on a scale in months, maybe even a year. Not knowing was bliss, right? Up to this moment, I was having an okay kind of day. I was looking forward to the conversation with the doctor and how wonderful life would be after the procedure. Then I saw my weight on the digital scale in what felt like billboard-sized font. *Did someone punch me and knock the breath out of me? Am I about to pass out?* I hadn't weighed anything near that since I was about to give birth to my last child. *How could this have happened? How could I have let it go this far?*

Finally.

I reached a number I couldn't live with.

This realization was so painful that it began the most important change.

It was my catalyst.

I was angry, furious really. I couldn't tell you at that moment what I was angry about, but what I know now is anger is a mask for fear, and I was scared. Scared I was out of control. Scared I was going to die early. Scared I was going to experience self-inflicted medical complications or diseases. Ted was working on a medical-surgical floor at the hospital, which was usually filled with diabetic complications. I knew I didn't want to end up on his floor and lose my toes, my eyesight, or have neuropathy simply because I wouldn't take care of myself. *Why would I not take care of myself? What could be more important?* Even if I were to say something like "my kids," I still needed to care for them. While nothing changed immediately, I assure you this moment on the scale was the wakeup call that started it all.

The doctor came into my room, and I was a mess. I couldn't stop crying. I tried to explain to her that I was not usually this overweight. I said things like, "I don't know how this happened," and "I don't know why it is so high." She compassionately nodded and let me get everything off my chest then, we discussed what I needed to know to prepare for the ablation.

One of the things was bloodwork. I hadn't had that done in a while and I kind of didn't want to know. *What if it said I had diabetes? I hate needles and don't like the sight of blood.* I couldn't do that. I was praying the type of prayer you pray when you let God know you're going to get serious about stuff if this will work out well. I was not yet diabetic, but my A1C was still elevated in the pre-diabetic zone.

Since we had been monitoring my thyroid numbers for a little while, it was determined that I, in fact, did have Hashimoto's disease, which meant checking my thyroid numbers a couple times a year to ensure I was getting the proper dosage of medication and support. I could usually tell when things were off. I would either start losing hair or have an extended period of not being able to sleep while feeling exhausted. Fun times.

The ablation went smoothly, and within a few months, my iron levels were breaching the normal range. What a difference this made. I finally had some energy and felt so much better. This gave me some mental space I desperately needed to even consider what I could physically do now that I was feeling alive again.

MORE MOTIVATING FACTORS

As if seeing my weight on the scale that day wasn't enough, there were other motivating factors to begin, and one of them was my children. One night, one of my daughters showed me her homework assignment from school. It was one of those "get to know my family" kind of worksheets. She had drawn Ted and me along with her siblings and dogs and then answered some questions about us. Next to "Mom" it said, "Favorite Meal." I was sure this was her teacher's judgey way of finding out all the dirt about the class moms. My daughter put down "Grapes, Chips, and Cheese." While that was (and sometimes still is) true, it was embarrassing. I felt ashamed that she told her teacher that was my favorite meal. *What am I, a five-year-old? Someone with no concern for their health?*

While those accusing thoughts ran through my mind, this hard glimpse in the mirror was another important motivating factor. I didn't want that to be what my kids thought of when they thought of me and how I ate. I wanted to be a better role model than that. I knew our families' histories. On Ted's side, obesity ran rampant, especially among the women. The same on mine. While our son may not face the same issues, as he is very tall and lean, he would have to face the choice of eating to feel good and have energy or eating and feeling lethargic and sluggish. The evidence was stacking up so that I had to make a change, and soon, before my bad habits became their bad habits.

Another motivating factor was my back pain, which was at an all-time high then. It hurt chronically. *How could I even think about exercising (the only way I knew or wanted to lose weight up to this time) with the pain so bad?* When I reached my bed at night, I was in tears. Life was bustling. I didn't have time to be in pain. There were kids' activities, church activities, and social gatherings, much less traveling I wanted to do, which the pain was prohibiting.

I finally reached out to my doctor and was prescribed physical therapy (PT) three times a week for an hour each time and homework of thirty to sixty minutes of more exercises. I'm pretty sure there was a quick mention in the conversation with that doctor about how losing some weight would probably help as well. This PT stuff felt like an additional part-time job with so many hours of driving, appointments, and homework. I didn't have time for all this. One of the most sobering quotes I came across was this:

> If you don't make time for your wellness, you will be forced to make time for your illness.
>
> **JOYCE SUNADA**

I didn't realize how much time, money, and energy I spent on my illness. It didn't dawn on me that I could flip the script and invest in my wellness, which I know now is much more fun. Despite the pain, I still had to keep going, which meant traveling to speak occasionally. I remember, like it was yesterday, the flight I took where I couldn't physically buckle the seatbelt on the plane. I tried and tried and tried. I started sweating from the embarrassment and exertion I was putting out to avoid the humiliation I was about to face. I reluctantly pressed the call light, and a flight attendant came over. She was polished, fit, and beautiful, possibly my worst nightmare of someone helping me fix this. *Is she going to judge me and give me a look of disgust as I ask her for a seat belt extender? Jesus, take me now,* I thought to myself. Thankfully, she was very kind and gentle and discreetly delivered the extender to me.

I sat through that flight looking down at my body and felt sad. Changing felt impossible. The mountain I would have to climb to be healthy was too high. I had tried climbing it before and always failed. I would get so far and then roll back down leaving a bigger mess than before. My body confidence was so low because I had made no investment in caring for it. I wasn't going to be someone who faked confidence because that was the movement at the time. While I do think people deserve love at any size, the bigger we are, the more our health is at stake.

One of the final motivating factors (you'd think I would have enough by now) was when I was helping create a slideshow for a church presentation. I had access to the church's photo files and was sorting through them and came across a photo of me that I hadn't seen before. At first, I was like, *Aww, a cute maternity picture of me.* Then I realized, I WAS NEVER PREGNANT IN TEXAS! Yet, in this photo taken several years into our time in Texas, I looked full-term pregnant. *Who let me leave the house looking like that?*

I was disgusted. I couldn't look at it but also couldn't stop looking at it. I was frozen. My abdomen, my arms, my face, all of it. How? I can honestly say I hated that person. I didn't need anyone else's help; I ripped her to shreds in my mind and felt nauseous when I was done. I downloaded that photo to my computer and buried it. If I ever needed to remind myself of how gross I was, I could open that file and inspiration was there.

Chapter Seven

Discontent is
the first necessity of progress.

THOMAS EDISON

Chapter Seven
A ROPE OF HOPE

It was about this time when I received a call from a caring friend in Nashville. She was a nurse practitioner and a former hair client of mine who knew my struggles and offered sound advice and transparency through the years. She told me about a weight loss protocol she learned about and had seen several friends and patients have success with. *Was this the thing I needed? Was this my turning point?* Ted and I listened and decided it was worth a shot. I told them both I was desperate and nearly hopeless, but the pain (in all areas) was enough that I was willing to try.

What intrigued me (and almost excited me) was how strict this program was. *After all, I deserve to be "punished" and put in food jail for how far I had let myself go. I should be whipped into shape. This will be hard, and that's what's coming to someone as disgusting and bad as me.* (I share these very real thoughts with you so you can see how my mindset changed over time.)

This program had a supplement to help me feel full, a supplement to give me energy, a lean protein powder (that became a meal sometimes), drink powders, liquid vitamins, and others I can't remember along with a carb-cycling meal plan that told me exactly what to eat and when. We were allowed one meal a week that was a cheat meal but were warned to not go too far off the cliff. This one miracle meal was supposed to allow us a break to crush a craving and create some caloric "confusion." All in all, this program was around $500.00 for a ninety-day supply. Not too bad, but not exactly sustainable in my mind at the time. After all, none of that included the cost of food but rather the supplements.

I carefully thought out when I wanted to begin this rigid plan and decided we should wait until after our son's birthday so I could have "one last dessert." Ted was going to do the eating plan with me, but not the supplements since he didn't need to lose that much.

On July 12, 2017, we took "before" photos, weighed in, measured ourselves, and began. Ted only needed to lose about twenty pounds. I was aiming for one hundred! Why not? I wanted to do it fast, and this was going to be the way. We were told to not weigh in for nine days so our progress could be wildly evident, and we followed the rules to a T, so if for some reason it didn't work, it wouldn't be our fault.

The first several days were rough. Between headaches from sugar withdrawal to not knowing what to do with my hands when they wanted to grab food, I kind of wanted to sleep but couldn't because I still had a family and a business to run. No doubt, major change like this also comes with a level of "change anxiety." Because this was about a 180° turn from the direction I was going, it had some change exhaustion to it. Nothing was the same as before, which is often a hard change to make and sustain long-term.

This new plan was like "cue the baked chicken breast, steamed broccoli, occasional brown rice, and apple" hamster wheel, and we were rolling with it. Yes, these foods in these portions guaranteed success for weight loss, but what about after that? I knew from all the years and diets past that I would need to keep the weight off the way I lost it, and this bland sadness wouldn't cut it for long. After the initial nine days, we saw fantastic results. I think I lost somewhere around thirteen pounds. *Wow, okay. Maybe I can eat this way for a little bit more.*

During this portion of my health journey, I didn't do hardly any exercise outside of easy walking and beginner yoga, which was mostly stretching. I was still nursing my back issues and felt too heavy or that I might hurt myself further. I also wanted to see how far I could get on diet modification alone.

We finished up the ninety-day protocol with great results. I was down around thirty pounds, and Ted was at his goal. I started to think about what this program was and wasn't. Yes, I lost weight. It fulfilled its commitment to me in that way, but it included products that weren't making me address the real issue—my relationship with myself. I was taking upwards of four to six products a day around the food to help me deal with the effects of eating less food. I didn't want this to be my life either. I could feel the, what I call, food pressure building and usually that meant I was about to jump, not fall, off the wagon, and that could get ugly quick. Bottom line—while it did help me lose weight, it wasn't sustainable.

FREEDOM TO SHIFT

Rather than quit and lose all the progress I had acquired, Ted wisely told me at the beginning of this "try" that if something stopped working, we would shift to something else that would. He even said we can shift as many times as it takes. Friends, I didn't realize how important this statement was. I had permission to try different things and find the way that best suited us. For me, this was more important because I believed the lie that I wasn't worth the money it took to try things. I believed I must find the best thing and stick with it. I had to give it my all, even if it meant suffering more because money had been spent (invested) in trying to help me get healthier.

This unworthy mindset was deep-rooted. I distinctly remember a conversation decades ago where my dad casually mentioned something like, "...and all the money we've spent on your mom trying to get her to lose weight..." kind of thing. I may not have it word-for-word, but the sentiment of a husband spending money on a wife over and over, trying to help her lose weight and being a burden, became engraved in my mind. *If I were to need this, my husband would have silent resentment towards me for being such an expensive problem.*

Until this conversation with Ted about having the freedom to shift, I assumed he already felt that I was a financial burden since I had vacillated between clothing sizes and programs several times. I assumed Ted felt the same about me as my dad did about my mom. I assumed Ted would get tired of me and hold it against me, whether he said it out loud or not. Hopefully, you can see the problem was me and me assuming everything. I had to get out of my way and overcome my limiting mindset. I must believe I was worth EVERY try.

A friend told me about a book written by a set of sisters who created a popular weight loss model. We decided to follow them for a few months as we were trying to figure out where we were going next. Their basic concept was carb and fat cycling but doing it on a meal-by-meal basis. If your meal had more carbs, it had to have low fat. If your meal had fat, it had to be low carb. I loved nearly all higher-fat meals and couldn't tolerate the taste of most of their high-carb meals in their popular cookbooks. I was able to lose about another ten pounds with this method and then sort of stalled for a little bit. What I discovered was, while no one is talking calories, you can easily consume more than your fair share when eating low-carb and higher-fat meals.

If the answer to making this program work for me meant eating more of those low-fat meals that didn't taste great (to me), it wasn't going to be the long-term solution. I do respect the program and see how it can help many people. Their focus is on nourishing your body while finding healthful substitutes for real cravings. While they did offer some of their own proprietary baking ingredients that are not required but helpful,

I did like that their program was largely food based rather than supplements.

Their overarching goal was to get you to where you could intuitively eat and sense when you were full without telling you exactly what a serving size was. This was also something I wasn't ready for at the time. I was only about six months to a year in and still very much white knuckling every meal. I didn't have the skills or mindset to self-regulate yet. While this program was worth the try, it wasn't the one. I remained with this model for about a year. I wasn't mad that the weight loss had stalled. I was happy that I was maintaining. Maintenance seemed to be the lost art none of the diet programs taught that I had seen. Maybe because I never got to that point or maybe they had a business built on people needing to lose weight.

TIME TO ADD ON

I had set up this benchmark of forty pounds as a place I would reintroduce exercise into my regimen. I was feeling so much better, my joints were hurting less, my confidence was growing—it was time to add on. One of my personal inspirations for this phase of my health journey was a college friend who started hers a few years before me. I was able to watch her lose and keep the weight off and see her start a fitness routine to compliment her nutrition changes. She would post about which online trainer's workout she did that day and the number of calories she burned. It was astonishing. I decided to use the same online platform since there was such variety, and I could press play on my television or device and stream the workouts anywhere.

I love to exercise and love variety. Sweating from exertion is one of the best feelings for me. Give me the burn. I printed accountability charts and felt complete satisfaction every time I marked off a workout. I was doing it. I'd lost forty pounds. I'd started working out like a beast and feeling stronger every day. This was my zone. After a few months, this zone became a slippery slope again. I started rationalizing eating more calories because I did a "hard workout." I would say things like, "I can add a second workout and burn this off."

I began relying too heavily on my workouts and laxing on the food side of things. I believed to my core, like many people, I could outwork a poor diet because I was somehow making it work. I could do strenuous exercise for ninety minutes or so a day and eat a lot more of what I wanted. Why wouldn't someone who loved to eat just exercise more? It made sense.

This worked until I tweaked my back and had to bench myself for a couple of weeks from the high intensity (read: mega calorie burning) stuff and saw the weight creep back on. My back got better, but then because I was overtraining, I injured my groin. Apparently, you need your groin for everything, so I had to take a major break for that as well. While I was still down with injury, I yo-yoed up and down, playing with the same ten pounds for a while. I will tell you, on a long-term health goal it is normal and healthy to take breaks from the weight loss phase. My body needed a break. My brain needed a break. I see now this is probably more of what was happening than anything else. It was a healthy pause that I could build from later and build I did.

I gave myself a solid six-month break from weight loss and then knew it was time to refocus and get those ten pounds off and see where I could go next. From these recent experiences, I knew I needed to continually search for sustainable change. I needed balance, so I took a more balanced approach to both eating and exercising in this next phase. I needed to further change my view of food to that of fuel rather than fun or rewarding.

Finding and valuing balance was a big part of my journey. I had held onto an extreme, all-or-nothing mentality that was sabotaging me. Anything I did had to be hard. It had to be perfect. It had to be above criticism (mostly my own). It had to be impressive to me. It had to scream commitment. It had to be hard enough to show people I wasn't tolerating this weight anymore. I was working like it had to come off instead of caring for my body enough to give it time to change. Appreciating everything it had done for me, my body didn't deserve the horrible treatment I was giving it.

This new quest for balance brought with it a micro shift in patience. I started to embrace the "it's not a race" mindset and an appreciation for how far I had come. I now had less of a grip on my timeline and more of an open hand with what progress followed. It felt like I had taken a small step off the hamster wheel or wasn't running so hard, which was a new feeling for me.

BUCKLE UP

I had an event to travel to, which sometimes brought anxiety. "What's the food situation?" was always my top-of-mind concern. It was difficult leaving the safety of my own home and kitchen stash and traveling while still in a "wet cement" phase. I packed a few grab things like protein bars and stevia-sweetened chocolate but had to trust there would be options for me. I tried to keep my worrying to a minimum, but each meal felt like a gauntlet.

My bag was packed, and Ted drove me to the airport. I boarded the plane, got my stuff situated, buckled my seatbelt, and pulled the loose end so it fit snugly. *Wait, what? What just happened?* I hadn't had a loose end on a plane seatbelt in a long time. I had nearly six inches of strap dangling! I know because I took a picture of it and shared it with Ted.

I couldn't believe it. This was one of the first tangible pieces of evidence of real change. I didn't need to make the embarrassing call to the flight attendant. I didn't need to secretly add an extender. I felt normal for the first time in a long time. I felt something else I hadn't felt in a long time or maybe ever—proud of myself.

This seatbelt experience translated into the confidence I needed to finally pull the trigger on a long-held dream of a family trip to Walt Disney World®. I thought, *If I can fit in a plane seatbelt now, I can probably fit all the rides and not have to get off a ride because I didn't fit or couldn't buckle.* We had saved for nearly five years for this trip, and I was excited to plan it. I was in the best shape of my post-childbearing life with plenty of energy to take on the long and strenuous days. In mid-February 2020, we set out to Orlando, excited for the upcoming adventure.

This trip was a major non-scale victory (NSV) for me. I fit on every ride comfortably and knocked the tens of thousands of steps out each day with the rest of them. I planned my splurges but looked for ways to eat what would make me feel great on such a special occasion. (Put a pin in this thought because I am returning to it.) We also packed our nutribullet* blender, ordered some simple groceries to our hotel room, and started each morning with a smoothie blend of fruits, veggies, and protein. This helped add fiber to the day and set me up for fewer cravings. Outside of the normal exhaustion, I felt so empowered. I tackled Disney like a champ.

Again, I was experiencing that newish feeling of being proud of myself. I distinctly remember pausing at one point and honoring past me for doing the work it took to get this far. This trip was a dream come true, and to be able to participate fully was a gift only I could give myself. It was no small gift either. By this point, it was two-and-a-half years of gifts in the shape of progress, courage, determination, overcoming challenges and setbacks, and continuing to show up.

THE REWARD CHANGED

Back to the pin, eating better because I wanted to was becoming a new normal for me. Until this point, food was the reward for good behavior or hard work. It was the comfort for anything stressful; the companion when I felt lonely. It was the thing I could look forward to in sad, hard, or dark times. I didn't see it while I was eating that way, but with greater awareness, I could tell that food was my main source of dopamine. It told my brain I could be happy, loved, feel appreciated and heard, and of course, validated. The struggles were real and to compensate for them, food was there to dull the pain.

The problem with this model is it was only rewarding "now" me or inner child me. It had no care or concern for the future me and was at odds with it. My inner child had no plans of growing up because that meant bland vegetables and sadness, or so I thought. The reward had to change. Feeling good must become more "exciting" (dopamine) than eating foods that weren't good for me all the time. Less joint pain must be the amazing indulgence. Fewer headaches, clearer skin, smaller clothes, and many more NSVs must become the rewards, and they did.

For most, if not all my adult life, I could only shop at plus-size stores. While I was grateful options increased dramatically over the last thirty or so years, I didn't know what it was like to have other options. I only shopped at one or two stores. One of my goals was to be able to fit in a brand of athletic wear that didn't currently offer expanded sizes. I remember the day I stepped foot inside the store, and honestly, I waited for a salesperson to approach and clarify their sizing or ask if I was lost or needed directions. When that ambush didn't happen, I meandered around the store, touching the fabulous fabrics, and seeing the cute designs that never ventured into the plus-sized world.

After a few minutes, a kind saleswoman came over and asked if she could help me. She was probably twenty and in stellar shape. I hesitated a little to share with her my feelings of imposter syndrome from being in the store but was somehow overcome with courage and spilled it all. I shared how I had lost all this weight and had only dreamed of being able to fit in these leggings that were far superior to the ones I had been struggling with and limited to.

She was so proud of me and shared how she helped her mother do the same. She felt very confident she could find me several options. I felt like *Pretty Woman*[5] in the fitting room with more options than I ever imagined. Since I wasn't finished losing all the weight I wanted to, I left with two fabulous pairs of leggings that I loved, knowing I would be returning for more in the future.

With my new leggings, workouts were even more fun because I looked forward to the incredible feel and fit with zero frustration. I had reached workout nirvana. With all this excitement, we decided to up the ante on our home gym and move it from our living room to the garage so we could push harder and sweat more. We installed a small television, and I continued streaming my workouts every day. Life was good.

THE UNEXPECTED

In March 2020, a couple of weeks after returning home from Disney World, everything shut down. COVID-19 was in full effect, and I don't know about you, but when it all seemed like it was crumbling down, I panic-ate like much of the American population. This was beyond stress. Not only was the whole world freaking out, but my husband was literally in the thick of it nearly every day for months as a nurse on the first COVID floor, and I was scared something would happen to him before they had any viable solutions.

I was home with our four kids plus our exchange student, who went from going to school every day to online school at home with no real plan or structure in place. It was a struggle. I continued working out but couldn't outwork my food intake once again. I gained around eight pounds, but thankfully, that trend slowed to a stop because of what Ted was seeing at the hospital.

Ted was among the first nurses to see COVID's effects on the community. One of the first things the medical community noticed was the part of the population being most affected. They were the diabetics, heart patients, lung patients, and the obese. It seemed those with health conditions (some of which were self-inflicted via poor health habits) were the ones succumbing to the virus.

This information scared me straight. I quickly saw that it was my responsibility to keep myself healthy so my body could fight any and everything going around. I cleaned up my diet with an even greater sense of mission and lost thirty pounds because of the lockdown. I was in great health and did not take it for granted. I also showed myself much gratitude for starting to care for my health years prior to this so I wasn't among the high-risk during this pandemic.

Chapter Eight

If you don't climb the mountain,
you won't see the view.

PABLO NERUDA

Chapter Eight
NECESSARY REPAIRS

All in all, from my starting weight in 2017, I was down seventy pounds. I couldn't believe it. I felt like an athlete on the inside but didn't quite look like one on the outside. One of the main issues with losing this much weight (along with multiple pregnancies) was excess skin, which for me created some serious problems.

I already had an undiagnosed skin condition that caused painful acne lesions, especially in areas where skin touched and trapped moisture and sweat. I had acne as a teen and young adult and assumed I was one of the lucky ones who had to deal with acne their whole life. Along with the lesions and heat rash, other complications arose, sometimes requiring antibiotics, powders, medicated cloth strips, and silver nitrate treatments, which were decently painful. To combat this condition, I showered daily, sometimes twice a day, to keep the problems at bay, but even with strict hygiene, I still had breakouts and painful rashes.

At one point, I had an abscess where the skin folded on my abdomen, which had to be treated with several different modalities. It was not only painful but cost time and money between appointments and medications. Not to mention, it affected my daily quality of life. I couldn't participate in any water activities with my family when it was in this state, which as Texans, was a regular occurrence for our family. Ted was concerned I could develop a wound, which meant hospitalization and extensive repair. I wanted relief because this was a source of sadness and sometimes depression. Here I was, doing all this work to get healthy, and the more weight I lost, the worse the skin issue became.

TAKING THE PLUNGE

Because of his extensive experience, Ted knew the cost of wound care and suggested before we get to that point, we consult with a local surgeon about skin removal. We met with an impressive doctor who explained the procedure and suggested we also address the bigger issue—diastasis (my abdominal wall situation). She echoed all the physical therapists from over the years and shared how repairing my abdominal wall would help alleviate much of my back pain.

During my consultation, she forcefully pressed her flat palm into my abdomen and held it there. I immediately noticed how much better my lower back felt from that temporary support. She told me that was what it would be like after the surgery. I couldn't believe it. I got teary-eyed because I hadn't felt that good in a long time. I couldn't remember life without back pain, I had to learn how to live through it and had been for years.

I shared with the doctor about my journey, mentioning something along the lines of how multiple pregnancies weakened my stomach muscles, and gently but honestly, she let me know that it wasn't only pregnancy but years of being overweight that caused my muscles to separate and push out rather than support my abdomen and spine. That wasn't what I wanted to hear by any means; nevertheless, I appreciated her candor. It increased my ability to trust that she would tell me the truth. I asked her if I was a good candidate for the surgery, and she said yes! I was a GOOD CANDIDATE!!!! Finally, all the years of hard work I had put in brought me to the precipice of one of the best rewards and solutions I could have dreamed of.

In addition to my back and skin issues, there was another painful component I'm sure many women can attest to after having numerous children, and that is permanently looking pregnant. No matter how many crunches or planks I did, no matter how much weight I lost, I looked six to seven months pregnant all the time. I couldn't wear dresses without someone asking me when I was due. I didn't even own a belt because where would I wear it? Over the bulge? Below the bulge? It hurt deeply every time I had to say I wasn't pregnant, sometimes multiple times to those persistent askers who didn't believe me.

I was ready to be done with these problems and now, I felt cautiously optimistic that I could trust myself to keep the weight off and stay in good shape to support the best and long-term outcome. Ted was supportive, my family was supportive, and even close friends I confided in were supportive. All of this was so exciting until I had to figure out if I was supportive and would consider permitting myself to get it done. This was quite the internal deliberation. There was the, *You don't deserve to be happy, it's selfish... This is too much money to spend on someone who didn't take care of themselves for so long like you,* side and the, *You've worked so hard and need this to get to where you want to go... You will feel unbelievable and be so glad you did this,* side, and it was all out war between the two.

While my rational side knew this was something I desired, my inner critic was holding me back. I tabled the idea for a while because my rational side wasn't strong enough at that time to fight for what it wanted. A few more skin lesions and rash issues later, and I was done. I was done lifting my flap of skin to clean and medicate underneath it. I was done with the pain of those sores. I was done with multiple showers a day to make sure I didn't have any breakouts from simply being hot since my last shower and sweating some. I was going to take the plunge and have the surgery.

PREPPING EVERYTHING

We looked at the calendar, knowing what recovery would mean, and decided January would be the best time to go for it. It would be cold outside, which would help mitigate the extra heat from all the compression garments I would need to wear for eight-plus weeks after. We scheduled the date, paid the deposit, and began working on the pre-op to-do list. It was nearly a daily battle to stay in the game. I kept imaging negative outcomes, including not surviving the surgery, and then I would have to talk with a friend or Ted to get my mind right again. I was riding the excited and terrified line for the months leading up to it. I'm sure I was a joy to be around.

I consulted a few individuals who underwent this lengthy and invasive procedure and asked for all advice as well as an account of their experience. I am so thankful I did because it helped set better expectations. One of the women advised me to get into the strongest shape I could beforehand because without my abs being able to work fully, every other muscle would be called upon to work more. I did exactly that. I focused on strength for the months ahead as well as eating well to accommodate what was coming. All my necessary bloodwork came back great, and I was given the green light to proceed. Yay…woah. The waves of excitement and terror crashed again.

The morning of surgery, we put the kids on the bus and headed to the surgery center where every step of the way, I was comforted, reassured, and double-checked to ensure everything would go smoothly. After confirming everything that was about to happen was correct, I was given a "top shelf" cocktail from the anesthesiologist and don't remember much of the day after that.

My next point of awareness or clarity was when I was in my private recovery suite hooked up to monitors. I wasn't totally lucid, but I remember it was getting close to evening from what I could see out my window. Ted was there for a bit before heading home to be with the kids. They wouldn't allow him to stay as they said he would need his rest to take care of me the following nights. While he was initially concerned, we were both relieved that I had my own private nurse to care for me through the night.

As I became clear-headed, I realized I was alive! Yay, major concern number one was out of the way. While I laid there still, everything was okay. The moment I thought about moving, I felt a considerable amount of pain and soreness despite the pain blocking medicines I was being given. Remember, I had four c-sections with my kids and knew what being cut open was like. This was much more involved and came with an extended recovery.

The work to correct the abdominal wall was what was causing the pain. I found out later that my abdominal wall was separated by over six inches, and the doctor had to "corset" those muscles back together. The skin removal part wasn't really painful at all. I was already numb in that area from all the c-sections anyway. I left the surgery center with a drain, which I was told would be in place for eight to ten days. Apparently, I am special and had mine for seventeen long days. This meant I couldn't shower for s e v e n t e e n days! I went from showering twice a day to no showers. Ted, my consummate helper and in-house nurse, took very good care of me even though it was somewhat humiliating to be sponge bathed as a grown woman.

Before my surgery, I had Ted put butcher paper over the lower portion of our bathroom mirror because I didn't know when I was going to be ready to see what I looked like and didn't want to get grossed out or pass out from the sight of myself. I imagined I might look like someone recently attacked by an animal (I have no idea where that came from, but I do know it was irrational). I couldn't even look at my drain. I didn't look down when Ted was sponge bathing me. I didn't want to know. I honestly assumed I wouldn't like what I saw.

Between the muscle relocation and the compression garments I had to wear, I needed to adjust things like breathing (at first) and eating. One benefit I didn't know or hear from anyone I talked with was that the muscles being where they should be made me feel fuller faster. Something was pressing on my stomach now and didn't give it much tolerance for overeating. It felt like I got the major pro of weight loss surgery without any of the cons I was concerned about. Everything felt tight, in a good way. There wasn't the puffiness or jiggliness. I could tell my back would feel much more support once I could stand up straight again, which was week one's goal.

After that amount of repair and rearrangement, my abdominal wall was extra tight, which caused me to be in a hunched position until I could lengthen the muscles into their new normal. This process took small daily steps of courage because not only was I sore, but also mildly terrified I might rip or tear something. The doctor told me I had a very thin abdominal wall and was surprised I didn't present with multiple hernias. *Good to know,* I thought.

WHAT DID I DO?

Meanwhile, I had to convince myself to stretch and attempt to lengthen these taught, sore muscles and not let fear get the best of me and derail my recovery. I worked diligently every day doing small micro stretches while resting and following the protocols. All was going well until about day four or five. I had buyer's remorse.

I felt trapped in my body because of how tight everything felt. I had a mid-level anxiety attack because I was used to having such great flexibility and mobility, and I wasn't sure I would ever get that back. I couldn't take deep breaths, and it was freaking me out at times. I regretted spending the money and putting myself and Ted through the whole ordeal. Once again, I didn't feel worthy. Why was worthiness still such a struggle? I am not sure I know the answer even to this day, but I can tell you assigning worth to yourself is a muscle that must be developed and strengthened. Assigning worth is the fuel for balanced self-care.

It took me about a day or so to get over the buyer's remorse because, well, I didn't have a choice. I wasn't used to having to rest and "take it easy" at all, much less for a solid eight weeks. I had an abundance of time on my hands but couldn't do much with it, which for my productive personality was very challenging. It forced me to slow down. It forced me to allow Ted and our kids to step up and carry my portion of things for a while.

It gave me time to reflect on the surgery and how grateful I was for being on the other side and recovering well, all things considered. I had finally reached one of my biggest goals and had the courage to go through with it. At my one-week follow-up, I had to strip down to only the gown so the doctor could check everything out. Of course, a mirror was in the room, but was I ready to see myself? Ted helped me get all the layers of compression gear off and work to stand up straight in case I wanted to peek.

I tried to casually glance without being too obvious, but once I saw myself, I asked Ted, "Is that what I look like? Is that me? Is this real?"

I could not believe it. This was the first time I felt I looked like the athlete I saw in my mind. No more looking pregnant. No more painful skin infections, lesions, or heat rash. Despite how tired my back was from working overtime to compensate for my abdomen, I could already tell it was going to be so much better.

I started to cry. I took a moment to mentally thank myself for doing it scared and going through with the surgery. I looked better than I could have ever imagined. I had a waistline again and could wear a belt or dress with no problem. My whole world was opening up. The weight of what was removed was way more than what showed on any scale.

My recovery continued on schedule, and after the initial eight weeks, I was permitted to add exercise back in. I was nervous about my stomach ripping open, but my doctor confirmed it would take a lot for that to happen. I worked back into things slowly and gradually but couldn't wait to experience workouts unencumbered by all that excess skin and diastasis.

By summertime 2021, I was back in my flow. All my flexibility returned and then some. I no longer felt trapped by the tightness as the muscles had lengthened properly to support my new normal. My back could feel the assistance of a properly functioning abdominal wall, and the range of exercises I could do expanded. Now, if anyone asks me, I always tell them I would do it all again in a heartbeat. It was totally worth it.

LIFE IN MAINTENANCE

For the next year, my goal was maintenance. My body had been through a lot, so I wasn't going to add an expectation of weight loss for a while. I wanted to see stability and regain some of the muscle I lost while recovering. Maintenance was something I had never practiced before. I was always on the way up or down from dieting, as were most people I knew. For anyone who has been involved in losing weight or needing to lose weight, I feel like the most mystifying part is maintenance. How do I stay where I've gotten? How do I balance healthy eating while occasionally incorporating treats like chips and queso (something I don't think I will ever quit enjoying)?

Around this time, I started following a registered dietician named Ilana Muhlstein on social media, whose approach to food made so much sense to me. It was logical. It was food-based, not product or supplement-based. What a novel idea! She wasn't only sharing from her wealth of knowledge and education, but she shared from personal experience, as she had lost over one hundred pounds herself and kept it off. I don't know about you, but having someone who has never experienced morbid obesity tell you how to lose weight never sat well with me. How could they possibly know what it's like, what I'm going through, how impossible it feels, etc.? I felt so understood by her.

She loves to eat a lot of food (volume eater). Same. She demands that the food she eats taste amazing. Check. She knows there always must be room for treats she enjoys; otherwise, it won't be sustainable. Wow, it's like she knows what I am thinking. As a former veggie hater, she helped me fall in love with new vegetables and new ways of preparing the ones I already ate. I also learned delicious substitutes for things I would crave that helped me satisfy the craving as well as stay on course with my goals.

I bought her book, *You Can Drop It* [6], and loved how simple her plan was. It is still something I think about when planning my meals. Some of the takeaways I had were about my relationship with food. What was I using food for? What did food do for me? How often did I try to make food the solution or the medication for problems it could never solve or cure? How much faith did I have in food that I expected so much from it? There are times I have a craving for something specific and now see how a stressor in my life pressed that button. Maybe I missed a relative that passed years ago, someone hurt my feelings deeply, or life felt out of my control, so let me eat something because I can control that.

Taking some time here to objectively analyze your own eating patterns will be some of the best investing you do for your health. You are not a robot. If you have tried one of those very strict, every meal planned for you, no cheating type of diets, what happened when you had the first bite of something off plan? How did you feel? Maybe relief, failure, pleasure, disappointment, the thrill of rebellion, like you should never have believed you could be successful? I have done it and seen it over and over again.

Because of all those strong feelings, it is difficult to make the next right choice because we don't feel worthy of making it. Our self-talk goes to garbage, making it nearly impossible to right the ship. The secret to maintenance is making a little bit of room for the things you want or "wish you could have" along the way. I try to decide my treat of the day by lunch, so I know what I can look forward to. And when it comes time to eat it, I can enjoy it. Make no mistake, over-treating is not the same. Whether it is number of treats or portion size of one treat, you must consider how it affects your overall goals.

METRICS

One of the points of data I look at every day is the scale. I know some have a negative relationship with the scale, but one thing about it is it gives unbiased feedback of one singular metric. In any health journey, there are numerous metrics to track, and weight is simply one of them. Once you separate your weight from your worth, this scale feedback becomes more neutral and less of a negative. Because I track what I eat, I can see how all of it affects my weight over time. It's not always the next day, in fact, many times it is the second day I see things more clearly.

The longer you go between weigh-ins the less accurate your data will be. This data is not used to punish me but rather to inform and optimize my decisions. I have become less afraid of weight fluctuations because of the years of daily data I have gathered. I have seen the scale go up over three pounds in a day and back down over the next two days. I have seen the scale stay the same for over a week when trying to lose. I have seen the scale drop two pounds even after a week of not eating super clean. The reason is food isn't the only factor.

One of the metrics I am now paying more attention to is sleep. Getting enough sleep is crucial for weight loss and overall health. I hadn't paid attention to this correlation until the fifth year of my health journey, and it is painfully obvious. Sleep not only affects our ability to heal and recover, but it also affects our choices the next day. When I am tired, what I am going to reach for, versus, when I am rested? We make better choices with the proper amount of sleep. For someone who has struggled with quality sleep for nearly a decade, this is something I must be even more intentional about.

Outside of food intake and sleep, there is the joy of hormones and how they impact the scale. I know from the data that my weight will go up and down no matter what I eat during my cycle. I am no longer surprised or upset with myself when this happens because I know it is a force out of my control. I also know that there are certain times within my cycle when my body needs a few more calories, so to deprive it of that would be a mistake.

LEARNING TO TAKE CARE OF ME

Let's not forget stress. Stress impacts our cortisol level, which is part of our blood sugar regulation. In short bursts, elevated cortisol isn't a very big deal, but long-term or chronic stress can tax the body systems it impacts. When looking at my health and weight loss, I always look at what my stress level has been and take that into account when analyzing my progress. Our family had an extremely difficult year a little while ago, and I took the time to honor my body for allowing me to maintain my weight for that year. I thanked it. That may sound crazy to you, but gratitude goes a long way. We give it to everyone else; we can give it to ourselves.

Some of my other favorite metrics are how clothes fit, overall strength, mobility, energy, photos of me, and how proud I am of myself. As any of those go up or down, I do my best to be curious and evaluate honestly. I take better care of myself by giving myself more opportunities for these to improve daily.

Chapter Nine

Your relationship with others
gets so much better when you
improve the relationship
with yourself.

ILANA MUHLSTEIN

Chapter Nine
REFLECTING

GRACE

At each stage of this process there have been opportunities to reflect on how I got here. I realized for years I held unforgiveness against myself, against my parents for not teaching me about food or making vegetables taste good, against skinny people in general, against the coach from high school, etc. For so long, they were my excuse for being the way I was. It was their fault and our society's. Why does society put so much emphasis on being skinny anyways? All through high school, I was on the studio art track and would envy the women in the paintings who were celebrated and esteemed as beautiful with all their rolls and chubbiness. Why was I born too late for that movement? I could have been awesome back then.

I reflected on why I was so critical of myself. It was as if I thought the more I tore myself down, the more I would want to change. Nothing could be further from the truth. It was around this time that I read one of the most powerful quotes I have ever come across:

> You can't heal a body you hate.
>
> **DR. WILL COLE**

Wow. I had been doing it all wrong. I had to start loving myself enough to change. I had to pour into myself, so I could have enough strength to continue in the direction I wanted to go. I had to believe in myself and let the details work themselves out. Instead of viewing workouts as punishment for all the bad eating I had ever done, I had to start viewing them as a celebration of what my body could do. Instead of pushing myself to work out every day (because I had to make up for so many years of bad habits), I had to learn to incorporate rest days. That doesn't mean laying around; it means letting my muscles heal and repair so they can do better the next day.

Instead of looking for opportunities to be critical of myself, I started looking for ways to honor and appreciate all effort applied, brave steps taken, and grace extended when I missed the mark. Grace seemed to be the next theme I needed to walk in for real growth to last. I had to practice giving myself grace when I needed it. This wasn't a blank check to do horrible things; it was more to help me reduce the burden of exhaustingly high expectations I placed on myself. Grace was to be extended when I tried to get everything in and done but didn't. Grace was there for me when our family faced the tough year, and it was all I could do to hold on and not end up curled into a ball in a corner somewhere. Grace helped me adjust my expectations to fit the season of life I was in, while still making health and care a priority.

This was a newfound freedom. I was no longer tightly tethered to perfection and rigidity, but instead, I was like a kite with more line to fly higher. I found that grace moved the needle more than criticism ever did. One of my favorite verses in the Bible is Romans 2:4, which so beautifully points out that God's kindness leads us to repentance. I had to learn this for myself and put it into practice so I could get the wounded, scared, defiant, rebellious, and often self-destructive me to come to the table for discussion.

MINDSETS I NEEDED TO CHANGE

One of the long-term assignments I unknowingly gave myself was to evaluate my mindsets more intentionally. Over the years, I took some time and starred in the metaphorical mirror, so I could be honest with myself and understand why I had a disordered relationship with food, myself, and other things. By no means is this a comprehensive list (it is always growing), but these are some that came to mind that might help you see yourself better as well.

Productivity: After denying it for a while, I finally acknowledged that I believed productivity was my main source of value or worth. The more I could produce or get done, the more value I had. This is a recipe for disaster. I felt like the hamster on the wheel who didn't know how to get off without a crash. There were only two options, go or go faster. Our pastor so graciously reminds us every so often that we are human beings, not human doings. I had to get to the place (and I'm still working on it) where I see value in myself even if I am not "doing" something all the time. I had to get comfortable letting other people pick up some slack. One of my personal mantras I've had to hold myself to is "ability doesn't equal responsibility." Just because I can doesn't mean I should.

Food Labeling: I know I'm not the only one, but foods were either bad or good; they weren't only food. Labeling foods in this way created an undesirable relationship with food. For example, if I wanted or craved bad food, I would then make myself feel shameful for wanting it. It was even worse if I *ate* the bad food. Heaven forbid. Or if I ate all good foods for breakfast and lunch, it was somehow permission to go off the rails for dinner. I now try to evaluate more of "how do I want to feel" when making food choices. For example, if I know I have a lot of work to do, it doesn't make sense to eat anything other than food that will give me energy and not make me feel sluggish. If I know I am going to a party, I plan for several treats and do not make myself think too hard about it. I do my best to eat in a way that I can be proud of, including indulgences.

All or Nothing: This mentality probably cost me years if not decades of progress and overall success. I was such a black and white thinker for so long that it sabotaged me repeatedly. On many of the diets I tried, I would do great if I made "perfect" choices. But as soon as I made a "bad" choice, it started a chain reaction of bad choices. Why didn't I see that one deviation didn't mean abandoning ship? One bad choice didn't have to mean a chain of bad choices. Along the way, I have realized that I can easily make the next choice a better choice in the right direction. I know, shocking idea. While this seems so rudimentary, it really was a life-changing revelation.

Never: This word should probably not be used regarding food. I used it a lot in the past with statements like, "I'm never eating fried foods again," "I'm never eating after 7pm again," "I'll never eat carbs again," or "I'm never having sugar ever again." Guess what? I have eaten and do eat them, but not in the same way I used to. Whenever I told myself never, it started this pressure cooker. I could withstand for a while and feel a certain amount of pride for doing so, but there were times when all I could think about was what I said never to.

After whatever amount of time, if there was any exposure or opportunity for the forbidden food and it was combined with a dip in resistance, it was the perfect time for the pressure cooker to pop and me to over-indulge. The inner child was demanding, and when I was tired or my will power was worn down all, I could do was give her what she wanted. I will say for me, saying "never" made me want it more. Something about it being taboo or "special" caused me to focus on it. I was trying to achieve addition by subtraction and that rarely works.

Deprivation is What I Deserve: You may have picked up on this theme throughout my story, but I wanted to highlight it here. This mindset twisted taking care of me into punishment. I focused on all the things I needed to remove from my life and deny myself because I felt unworthy of happiness, joy, and any other positive emotion that seemed too extravagant. I have found the more generous I am with myself, the better I respond.

I love rewarding myself with new leggings when I reach a goal. I love positively incentivizing myself rather than negatively because it makes me press into the challenge versus fear the challenge. I've learned there are two types of people when it comes to what motivates them, those motivated by the carrot and those motivated by the stick. The carrot is the positive reward waiting on the other side of achieving a goal. The stick is punishment or negative consequence to metaphorically smack you until you reach the goal. I am definitely motivated by the carrot much more than the stick, so rather than deprive myself, I reward.

My Money's Worth: Oh man, one thing about honestly facing your food mindsets is it will make you face your money mindset. In the name of not wasting, I overate so many times. I felt I worked so hard for the money I made that I wasn't about to waste any by leaving food behind, even the cold bag fries. For some reason, taking any or all the meal home wasn't appealing, so the only solution was to eat it all.

Now, I have no problem only eating what satisfies me and putting whatever I want to revisit in a go box. I get to satisfy both my frugality and my health goals simultaneously, and that feels great. Most days, I can't complete a whole restaurant meal due to the large portions, so I plan to either cut it in half and box it up, share the meal with someone, or worst case, leave some behind. I now value my health goal more than my financial reasoning. It took me a long time to get here, but it is a great place to be.

I Don't Want to Hurt Their Feelings: People often give food as gifts, whether it is a cookie here or doughnut there. It's hard to say no when they are standing there waiting and watching you. Now, I don't mind taking the offer but will usually say something like, "I'm full now, but this might come in handy later. Thank you for thinking of me."

There is also the dinner invitation where we are welcomed into a family member or friend's home, and all cooking is out of our hands. I used to enter those engagements terrified because what if nothing served was healthy? What if it puts me way off my goal for that day? I would often eat at my own expense because I didn't want to hurt their feelings and didn't have a plan. One of the ways I overcome this obstacle now is I bring a veggie or fruit option or there is always a salad. Not a boring or sad salad, a beautiful and yummy salad for everyone to enjoy. Friends help friends eat veggies!

Bargaining, Rationalizing, and Special Permissions: A few examples of these slippery slopes went like this in my mind: "I worked really hard today, so I am going to treat myself to…," "I'm hormonal and just want…," "I've been good all day, I deserve a…," or "I did a hard workout. I earned some…" These don't even include eating out and how that became a treat every time because it was special or eating everything because I didn't want to waste money. While I am not saying food should never be a reward, I have worked hard to reduce the frequency and continue to search for and implement other things. Some of my favorite substitutions for food rewards are rest, some pampering like a foot massage or nail service, sauna time, a night off from cooking, game night, friend time, or simply a long shower and straight into comfy clothes.

Idolatry: Try to follow me here because this subconscious mindset I held might sound like an overstatement at first glance: food was an idol. Idol simply means "an object of extreme devotion."[7] I was devoted to food. I followed food around. I thought about food all the time and let food take the wheel for most of my life. This is hard to explain to someone to whom food isn't an issue specifically, but like any other negative addiction, it has the same destructive patterns and outcomes. I let food be more important than one of the most important things—my health. Without health, few other goals can be met, if any at all.

One of the key mindset shifts that had to take place was assigning a value (devotion) to what indeed matters. I had to stop wishing for change that required consistency and value what that meant in a long series of decisions. I had to value my choices enough to follow through and hold the line. I still must do this. In some respects, it gets easier with time, but the choices always present themselves.

Taking care of myself shows up most in the smallest decisions made consistently. It looks like putting on gym clothes and lacing up my shoes every day for some kind of movement or exercise. It looks like drinking a lot of water. It looks like going to bed on time as much as possible. It looks like taking vitamins and starting the day with a protein packed breakfast. When taking care of myself is the goal, there is no room for being a slave to or worshipper of food. Taking care of myself is a balanced mix of yes and no, now and not now, all with a healthy end in mind.

ONE OF THE BIGGEST NEEDS

There are plenty more mindset issues I've had to work through, but these are the ones that stood out to share in this book. If you don't deal with these, great. Don't think these are the only ones. This process has been about meeting one of the biggest needs I had—trust. I had to get honest with myself, and I still do. I had to acknowledge what felt like childish feelings to see progress in my mind, which translated into progress for my health. Until I disciplined my mind to line up with my goal, it usually worked against me. This discipline didn't come through motivation. It came through consistency.

I had to stop putting question marks on the ends of statements. I'll give you an example: "I'm going to the gym today?" No. Question marks had to be removed from the equation when it came to things I wanted to accomplish with my health. "I'm going to stay on track even though I am going to a birthday party where there may be wonderful food, including cake I want to eat?" No. I'm going to stay on track and decide what single outstanding thing I want to try and enjoy while sticking to what will make me feel great tomorrow.

I had to get to the point where I could trust myself because frankly, I didn't for a long time. I would say these ridiculous things like the "I'm nevers" and then ultimately break the promise. My brain would go, "See, I knew you weren't going to stick to it. You never do."

> ## Self-confidence is built by keeping the promises you make to yourself.
>
> **ED MYLETT**

Breaking trust with myself continually took a toll. It chipped away at my self-confidence. It undermined my desire to be healthy and take care of myself. If you've made it this far, you can imagine how many times I told myself I wasn't going to gain the weight back. And when I did, it usually came with even more weight due to the shame, disappointment, and destroyed self-confidence because once again, I couldn't trust myself. I had to shift my whole behavior. Instead of telling myself things I couldn't possibly live up to, I had to make different promises that were more attainable while still flexible like:

- "I am going to do my best to stay committed and make choices that reflect that."

- "I love the way health feels, and I want to give more of that to myself."

- "I want to be able to live as a blessing to my family and not a burden, so I will continue to exercise and do my part to ensure that."

- "I value myself and will make the daily deposits only I can make to retain and increase that value."

- "I know that health is wealth and will do what it takes to grow and protect it."

These statements and beliefs had to satiate both sides of me—the inner child with needs and desires and the adult who benefits from discipline and thoughtfulness. I had to make room for both fun and excitement, as well as long-term joy and fulfillment. What this looks like for me these days is eating eighty percent on track or "healthful" and twenty percent treats and splurges. Nothing is off-limits. Nothing is a bad food (except the few foods I can't stand, like tomatoes). Instead, the evaluation process looks like this:

- Where am I on the scale these days?

- What direction do I want to see the scale go tomorrow?

- How did _____ food make me feel the last time I ate it?

- Did I enjoy it?

- Was it worth it?

- What do I have coming up that I may want to set aside caloric space for?

- How do I feel about myself?

- What decision would make me feel even better?

I try to leave room each day for something I would consider a treat, whether it's some Lily's* dark chocolate baking chips in my Greek yogurt, Manchego, chips and salsa, or even fries. The main difference now is simply quantity. Reluctantly at first, I have become more aware of serving sizes and daily do better to stick to them than ever before. I also leave room for an indulgent meal each week. Previously, indulgent meals were much more frequent and took all the wind out of my progress sails.

One of the biggest "then and now" comparisons for me was seen on vacation to an all-inclusive. The first time I went was for our tenth anniversary. I had no boundaries. I ate and drank to get my "money's worth," and while there, there was a measure of enjoyment in that, but it gave me that slobbish, yuck feeling. I wasn't proud of myself, which was a feeling I undoubtedly longed for.

Fast forward to our twentieth anniversary at another all-inclusive, and things looked incredibly different. I exercised every day and participated in poolside dance classes and competitions. Breakfasts were proteins and beautiful fresh fruit. Lunches were veggies, proteins, and chips with fresh guacamole. Dinners were high-quality proteins with veggies and a small dessert treat. I stopped when I was content and didn't push myself into cleaning my plate if I wasn't hungry. I came home and was so proud that when I weighed myself, I had only gained three pounds, which I lost within two days of getting home.

Who was this new person? So confident. So free. I was able to enjoy myself *while* caring for myself. I was so proud of that balance of discipline and enjoyment. It was a victory, for sure. This was the result of huge amounts of trust built slowly over time. When every kind of food and drink was available, all the time, every day, I didn't have to turn into a feral animal and go nuts. I could be picky and only eat the things that were absolutely delicious to me. I could try new things or only get a bite of some while filling my plate with food that would help me stay on track. I celebrate this shift and am so thankful I put in the work to get there.

Chapter Ten

Example is not the main
thing in influencing others.
It is the only thing.

ALBERT SCHWEITZER

Chapter Ten
THE POWER OF INFLUENCE

TRYING NOT TO PASS IT ON

I also wanted to call this section "The Trickiness of Parenting While Trying to Change Your Family's Trajectory." As you may recall, one of the biggest motivators for me to begin was seeing that my kids were coming up on puberty, and I didn't want them to copy me or make the same mistakes I did and suffer the numerous consequences. Before I started, I would duplicitously make them eat vegetables even though I wouldn't. I wasn't yet strong enough or demanding enough to change myself, but I was bound and determined they would not follow in my footsteps or the generational habits.

More than anything, I wanted them to have the freedom, physical confidence, and strength to do whatever they wanted. I didn't want their bodies to hold them back as mine did me. Being active was of high value to our family. Our son was always in a sport and has found his passion in ice hockey. Our daughters participated in gymnastics year-round and then sports in their seasons. All four have found activities they enjoy, and I am very grateful because keeping them in motion generally hasn't been very difficult.

On the food front, there have been challenges because of my history. Once committed to my health, I cleaned the house out. If it was a dangerous food (meaning I didn't have the willpower to resist it at the time) it was gone. I went cold turkey and emptied our house of sugar, most processed foods, and chips and brought in the vegetables. While I don't think any of that was "wrong," it was a bit much for the kids to experience all at once and came with some unforeseen consequences.

Sneak eating became a very real thing. I would occasionally clean or help tidy their rooms and come across stashes of wrappers from candy, granola bars, crackers, and anything else they could get their hands on. I would get reports from fellow parent friends that our kids ate all their snacks as if they had never had them before. The parents thought it was comical; however, I was freaking out.

"Great, I've created sneak eaters," I would say to myself and judge every parenting choice I made. *How do I undo this? How do I help them understand that this behavior will backfire, and they won't like the outcome?* I had so many questions and had no grid for this problem. I thought removing access would be the solution, but I was wrong.

I had to honor their thoughts and feelings on the subject and, in some ways, violate my conscience to get there. I didn't want them to eat anything that would not be good for them, but that was an unrealistic expectation I could never meet or ever hold them to. It was setting us all up for failure. I must remember that I too was a picky eater and had to find my own way into trying, liking, and eventually loving vegetables.

I needed to extend them some slack and find moderation in what foods we had at home and allowed them to have. I needed to relax, or I was going to fuel a different eating problem in them. At various times, they would share that they felt I was judging every food choice they made. I was. I was driving myself nuts being so concerned with every bite they put in their mouths. This wasn't their issue, it was mine. I was terrified of passing obesity down to them.

I had to apologize and sometimes still do because I slip back into this unhealthy, overbearing mode. I acknowledged I didn't do this transition perfectly despite how hard I tried. I had to share with them the naked truth of why I cared so much. Several of my kids were so young when I began that they didn't even remember what I looked like before. They couldn't process it all until I showed them the before pictures. They didn't recognize me, much less remember me that way. I wanted their future to look different than the past I had, but the way I was doing it wasn't the way to get it done.

One of the things I had to adjust quickly is that for a while it wasn't likely serving one meal for dinner was going to be the best solution. Ted and I had to come to terms with the fact they weren't jumping on the bandwagon as fast as we thought, so adult dinner and kid dinner became a very real thing.

This way, Ted and I could eat optimally, and they could eat something they wouldn't complain about while still getting decent nourishment. Occasionally, the unicorn meal comes along that meets everyone's standards, and when that happens, we celebrate.

Another thing I had to set aside to reach my goal was "fewer dishes." When preparing two dinner meals and on the weekend sometimes two lunches, dishes pile up. Dishes used to be a big deterrent for me even cooking for myself. Now I try to not let making a mess be a factor at all. The mess can and will get cleaned up, and it isn't as big a mountain as I had made it in my mind.

NAME THAT FOOD

I also wanted to be sure our kids knew the main food categories and what purpose they serve. We regularly talk about getting enough protein, the purpose of fiber, healthy fats, and the time and place for treats, especially sugary ones. I remind them it is always best to not eat something sugary on an empty stomach, instead tack it onto a balanced meal at the end to help balance blood sugar levels. I try to have them aim for only one "dessert" a day, whether it is a soda, candy, cookie, or whatever.

Mindfulness around the quantity of sweet things is very important. I remind them they never have to finish a dessert, fries, or anything in the treat category. They can always set some aside for later that way they can fully enjoy it and not feel yucky. Believe me, most of the time this is just a suggestion. They are still kids who go through most of their day surrounded by the powerful marketing and presence of sweets and junk food.

As much as they will listen (which is very subjective), I try to educate my kids about food and the effects it can have on them both short and long-term. Along the way, I learned that type 2 diabetes is not hereditary. Because of all the medical forms at doctors' offices, I believed it was. When they ask the family history of type 2 diabetes, it isn't because it is something passed down in genetics, it is because we often become like those we eat around. Unless you make conscious decisions to be different, there are strong chances you will be influenced by those you eat around. As I said before, I didn't want my kids to copy my negative behaviors around food and health, so I knew I had to lead the change.

Besides type 2 diabetes, the other statistic that got my attention was the correlation between obese parents and children. If parents are overweight or obese, there is an eighty-nine percent chance their kids will be overweight. If parents are of healthy weight, there is a less than a one percent chance their kids will be overweight.[8] This statistic is staggering. As a parent, if nothing else inspires you to change your life, think about the lives of those around you who are watching and following. You are an influencer.

I have heard from my kids how hard it is to eat differently, especially while surrounded by friends who have junk-filled lunch boxes with stuff (notice I didn't say food) engineered to make them craved. I must agree with them. It is much easier to follow the pack, but as I say to them consistently, they have things they want to do and participation in them will be much easier if they feed their bodies well.

With as much information as I, my kids, or any of us have, for that matter, it is abundantly clear that information doesn't always lead to transformation. If it did, we would all be fit and rich. Much of the time, we love information. We get high on learning but then fail to act on what we've learned. Most of us would acknowledge we "know" how to eat healthily. We "know" what it looks like.

I used to think eating healthy meant the saddest meal of baked chicken breast and steamed broccoli all the time. I can't even with that meal. It looks like misery. For me to succeed, food still had to be fun, even if it was healthy. It had to be tantalizing visually and in taste. I promised myself no matter how many fitness people promoted the chicken and broccoli combo, I would not make myself eat anything I didn't like. While I love both those things, prepared in certain ways, if they aren't absolutely delicious when they are in front of me on my plate, I'm not eating them.

INFLUENCE MATTERS

For this reason, I do my best to keep inspirational health leaders in my social media feed as much as possible. Positive role models, experts who make health and wellness fun, fitness tips, and success stories are a few examples of ways I receive helpful "advertising" messages that keep me on track. I used to follow foodie influencers, watch cooking shows, shows where they visited greasy spoon restaurants, and talk about delicious, over-the-top concoctions, which are basically food porn. I wouldn't be hungry before I saw their post or video, but afterward, I would start foraging for something to quench that sparked desire.

Our behavior is largely based on influence. What *has* influenced us, what *is* influencing us, and what *will* influence us. While we did not have a choice on what influenced us as children growing up in households with certain behaviors around food, we can choose what we are influenced by now and in the future.

I had to look even deeper than social media and evaluate which people in my life were supporting my health goals and which were enabling my weaknesses. At the very beginning of this, Ted and I were hosting a weekly community group where we would all share a meal and play poker. I remember the first week Ted and I planned to make a shift in what we ate and served but still made the regular menu available. We made a tray of traditional lasagna and another tray where we subbed the pasta with sliced zucchini while everything else was the same.

I was honestly intimidated to make this change in front of friends I had eaten with for years. A few friends balked at the new option, but several tried it. Thankfully, everyone was positive about the change I was trying to make for myself. A few of the shifts we made while staying social were nacho night turned into taco salad night, a plate full of chips and dip turned into a few chips with mostly sliced cucumbers or mini bell peppers and dip.

I wasn't going to let changing the way I ate turn me into a hermit. I remember in diets past being terrified of eating out at restaurants with people or any kind of food-centered hangout because *what if I lose control? What if I go off the deep end or off the rails?* I can honestly say that practicing makes progress. Each time I can go out to eat or be in an "uncontrolled" food environment, I ask myself, what is the treat I want most here? Maybe this restaurant has a great dessert or marvelous cheese board I want to enjoy. I build the meal around the treat. I look for a salad with protein and perhaps trim off some of the heavier toppings, so I can leave room for a portion of the dessert. I also know I can eat some of the dessert there and take the rest home for another day and spread the treat out over time.

I also am very aware that I can still be influenced if I am feeling particularly weak (tired, stressed, emotional, hormonal, etc.). One strategy I learned from Ilana Muhlstein is to order first. Before you hear your friends' orders, get your solid choice in first. That way you don't cave based on the influence of other people's orders. Perhaps your order might positively influence someone after you? Who knows!

THE FLIP SIDE

I learned quickly that not everyone is happy for you when you decide to change your life. Why? Because progress provokes people who are not making or choosing progress. It forces them to reflect on their status and often creates a negative response. We know misery loves company, and when the company moves on to better things, misery becomes lonely. I had to remind myself their angst was not truly aimed at me. I was simply a reminder to them that they weren't yet choosing progress, and by not choosing progress, they were choosing to stay the same or digress.

I remember watching a college friend's health journey on social media. Daily, she would share her post-workout photo and Apple° watch details; occasionally, she would post how many pounds she had lost. I was provoked but not to anger. I was provoked into action. She was a big inspiration to me. Seeing her consistency, honesty, and vulnerability made me see I could make changes too.

One of the biggest reasons I have taken the time, cried the tears, faced stuff I didn't want to again, and shared the deeply personal details on these pages is to hopefully provoke you—not to anger but to action. To help you see that slow progress is still progress. Kindness is the best way to motivate yourself. Truth is the strongest foundation to build lasting change. I am so glad I gave myself one more chance. I had plenty of history of not keeping promises I made to myself, but that isn't where my story had to end. I could change. I could change my expectations from things having to be perfect to things being my best effort.

> Waiting for perfect is never as smart as making progress.
>
> **SETH GODIN**

I have taken the slow yet sustainable path to health. Maybe that doesn't sound exciting or impressive to you, but one thing I know you always look for when friends or family lose weight is WILL THEY KEEP IT OFF? As a serial dieter, nothing has been more impressive to me than keeping the weight off. When you give yourself patience, your body will respond. I no longer ban any foods or deny myself for long periods of time and then have a "cheat day," I find that the more I acknowledge the small desires of my inner child and treat her along the way, the less she actually wants to derail me. She only wants to be heard and validated.

Perhaps you have denied the part of you that wants the treats in diets past and have seen the repercussions of that in the pounds gained on top of the ones lost. I've been there. I've done it. I've learned from it. Take that information and put it to good use. Don't shame yourself for wanting those things. Find healthy ways to incorporate them so you don't build up pressure and end up on a binge. You are worth one more chance. You are worth forgiving for all the broken promises. Make better promises this time. Promise to keep trying. Promise to get back on the horse if you fall off. Promise to be honest with yourself.

Don't mistake taking care of yourself for being self-centered. Taking care of you IS taking care of your family. Taking care of you IS taking care of your friends. There is only one you, only one me, and our bodies are the vessels we steward. We have the choice to make our bodies a prison or a vehicle. I lived too many years with my body as a prison. I felt trapped, limited, and ashamed like a prisoner would feel. As I started to care for myself, the prison began turning into a vehicle to help me do the things I really wanted to do. I was no longer too big for rides, too heavy to walk long distances, or in too much pain to play with my kids. Every area of my life improved as my health improved.

It's never too late to begin. Of course, I wish I had made this decision years before I did. I try to tell anyone and everyone who will listen to make changes now, but I know what it's like to have someone try to make you do something you're not ready to do. But, when you are ready, go for it with all your might because your life depends upon it.

I've never seen a person who improved their physique and didn't start improving every other area of their life.

DR. JAMES DINICOLANTONIO

QUICK START GUIDE

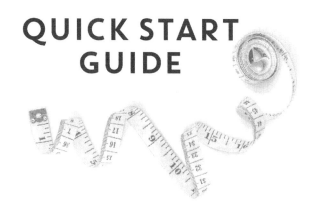

Here are some simple steps to getting started on your health journey today!

Get on the Scale—One of the biggest things you need is accurate information. The scale is one piece of information you will need for measuring progress. It is not the ONLY one, but it is a valuable one. The more points of data you gather, the better the information you will have to analyze what works and doesn't work for your body. I weigh daily because I love data.

Measurements—Knowing where you're starting helps evaluate how far you've come in the months and years ahead. I wish I had kept my initial measurements. I can't find them and kick myself regularly for losing them. Measure your right and left upper arms, thighs, and calves, as well as your waist and hips. Date each round of measurements. I usually measured every two months or so. You can do it after a certain amount of weight loss, like ten-pound increments.

Take Photos—Sometimes we can't "see" the changes in ourselves like others can as we work to dismantle the mental image we hold tight. Progress photos inspire me, especially when the scale doesn't move how I want it to. I still have my "day one" photos and regularly go back and thank that woman for being brave and strong enough to make these changes.

Start with One Change—Pick one thing you can change right now and stick with it. Maybe it's drinking a glass of water first thing in the morning. Maybe it's switching breakfast from cereal to scrambled eggs or something more protein-rich to help set you up for a fabulous day. After two weeks of consistency, add in the next small change. This isn't a race.

Keep the Goals Small—When facing a mountain of changes that need to be made, it is easy to become overwhelmed or feel it isn't possible. This is like trying to eat the elephant all at once. We know it won't work. Set small, attainable goals and then celebrate every one. I didn't wait until I lost fifty pounds to be excited. I was excited about every single one. I celebrated going down a size. I celebrated being able to hold a solid plank for thirty seconds. I celebrated every time someone commented on my weight loss. Small goals mean many celebrations. That's my kind of party.

Know Exercise's Place—What took me years to accept was that weight loss is upward of eighty-five percent food related and fifteen percent exercise. I wanted it to be the other way around. I love exercising but hated vegetables when I started this whole thing. Now, I know and have accepted food is the lever that moves the scale, and exercise is what changes my body's strength, shape, and function. You may have heard this saying, "You can't outrun a bad diet," it is the truth. There is not enough time in the day to try and correct the caloric damage of a bad diet through exercise. Not only that, but our bodies also need time to recover. It would be an endless, unsustainable cycle. Exercise drastically improves the quality of your life but isn't the main lever to change your weight.

Evolve—Each year, I reevaluate my goals and establish new goals. Some years, my goals aren't even weight related. For example, this year's goal is to increase my flexibility to do the splits. Another goal is to be able to dead hang for a minute. A big goal, which may take longer than a year, is to be able to do a pistol squat. If you don't know what that is, look it up. Getting your health in order will likely lead to other changes in your life, like better boundaries, healthier relationships, going for promotions, and taking leaps of faith because you have built yours up and know you can do hard things.

I would rather be the master of my
wellness than a slave to illness.

CHARITY BRADSHAW

A NOTE
FROM ME TO YOU

I believe in you. I believe you can begin again, and I trust you will do better this time. I know it will be hard. I know your progress will not be a straight line. I have faith that you will reach a point where the pain of staying the same will become too much to bear, and you will get out of your comfort zone and reach for your health with all your might. You will forgive yourself when you relapse into old habits. You will give grace to those around you who are not changing with you. You will begin enjoying the rewards of caring for yourself and finding ways to increase those regularly.

You are worth it. You are worth every dish it takes to cook a beautiful, healthy meal. You are worth every substitution request at a restaurant that helps you stay on track. You are worth the time it takes to prepare for a week of breakfasts, lunches, and dinners. You are worth the money it costs to join a gym or find a fitness community. You are worth every tear you will cry as you tear down walls and build your health empire.

I hope you have taken everything I've shared through a filter of love because that is how I wrote it. Immense love, grace, patience, and everything else it has taken me to get to where I am today. Feed yourself these things and watch yourself flourish. Your best days are ahead!

Much love and belief,

Charity

DID YOU ENJOY THIS BOOK?

Help us get this powerful message in front of others who need it!

Here's how:

- Write a positive review on your favorite online book retailer's website.

- Buy a copy for a family member or friend.

- Post a picture of you and this book on social media and tag Charity in it.

FB—@charitybradshawINC

IG—@charitybradshaw

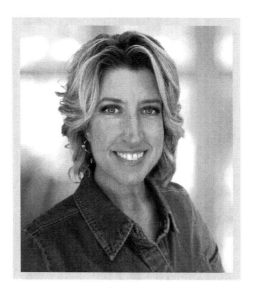

ABOUT THE AUTHOR

Meet Charity Bradshaw, a passionate author, public speaker, and entrepreneur who embraces her calling to inspire and uplift others. Her writing career began with the encouragement of her mother, Joan Hunter, who recognized Charity's immense wisdom and insight and insisted she share them with the world. Despite Charity's initial concerns about being too busy as a devoted wife, mother to four children, and running her own businesses, her mother's persistence prevailed, and Charity began penning the messages placed in her heart.

As an author and speaker, Charity focuses her passion on empowering others to embrace and nurture their unique gifts and activate their true purpose in life. She wholeheartedly believes every individual has untapped potential waiting to be unleashed. With her compelling words, Charity encourages her audience to shed their self-imposed limitations and step into the greatness they were divinely designed to achieve.

Charity also offers a transformative twelve-week course called "Launch Author Coaching" where she guides aspiring writers on how to draft their books with excellence. Additionally, she runs her publishing company, LifeWise Books, ensuring that remarkable stories find their way into the world.

In her personal life, Charity shares a beautiful journey with her best friend and husband, Ted, who she has been married to since 2002. Together, they are raising their family in the Greater Houston area of Texas. When not pursuing her passion for writing and speaking, you can find Charity at her happy place—the gym—where she builds community, balance, and strength. She dreams of one day having a personal chef to create delicious and healthy meals that complement her goals. After all, a dreamer can dream, right?

Through her inspiring words and unwavering commitment to help others, Charity Bradshaw continues to impact lives and encourage people to embrace their full and true potential.

www.charitybradshaw.com

Additional Resources
FROM CHARITY

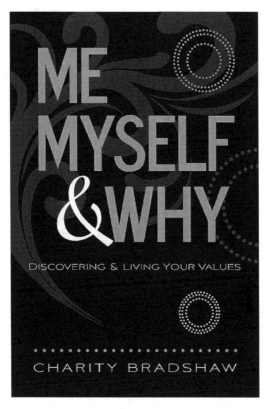

ALIGN YOUR TIME

Many of us have said "yes" to things to please our family, friends, boss, or others which has created a life and schedule we resent and barely survive in. This book will help you evaluate how you spend your time so you can better align yourself to how you were designed to function in this world. Reduce stress by intentionally editing what's on your plate to make room for things that bring joy, peace and fulfillment.

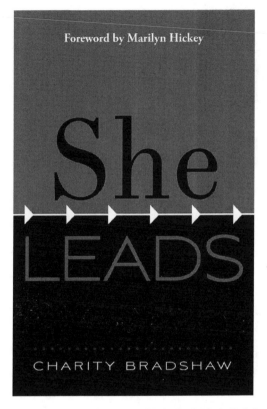

GO BEYOND ORDINARY

Leadership is not relegated to a certain age, gender, degree plan, or economic status. We all possess gifts, talents and ideas that equip us to serve and lead from right where we are. This book will inspire you with examples of women who took their ordinary life and became extraordinary by offering their unique self to the problems they encountered. Through their stories, we can all be encouraged to take what we have been given, live beyond ourselves, and make an impact.

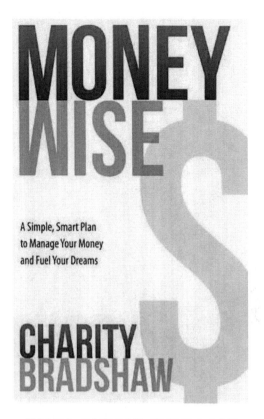

FUEL YOUR DREAMS

Money isn't simply something we use to pay the bills; it is a catalyst for nurturing our aspirations. Our financial choices unveil our true desires, often pitting immediate pleasure against long term goals. This book simplifies financial organization, empowering you to chase your God-inspired dreams. Learn saving tips, reshape your money mindset, and step confidently toward your destiny.

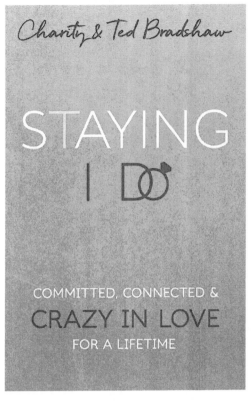

Charity & Ted Bradshaw

STAYING
I DO

COMMITTED, CONNECTED &
CRAZY IN LOVE
FOR A LIFETIME

IN LOVE FOR A LIFETIME

One of the most important and longest relationships you have is with your spouse. Many couples invest months or even years planning their wedding, but often neglect planning for their marriage. Beyond the honeymoon lies a life together and it is worth the work. Ted and Charity Bradshaw openly share the principles that have enriched their marriage, making it warm, fun, and fulfilling, regardless of the challenges they've faced. Whether you are a nearly married or a seasoned couple, this book will motivate you to strengthen your relationship even more.

ENDNOTES

1   "Stewardship Definition & Meaning." *Dictionary.Com*, www.dictionary.com/browse/stewardship.

2   Scripture taken from The Message: The Bible in Contemporary English, copyright©1993, 1994, 1995, 1996, 2000, 2001, 2002. Used by permission of NavPress Publishing Group.

3   "Body Dysmorphic Disorder." *Mayo Clinic*, 13 Dec. 2022, www.mayoclinic.org/diseases-conditions/body-dysmorphic-disorder/symptoms-causes/syc-20353938.

4   "A1C: What It Is, Test, Levels & Chart." *Cleveland Clinic*, my.clevelandclinic.org/health/diagnostics/9731-a1c.

5   Marshall, Gary, director. *Pretty Woman*. Buena Vista Pictures Distribution, 1990.

6   Muhlstein, Ilana, and Lisa Lillien. *You Can Drop It!: How I Dropped 100 Pounds Enjoying Carbs, Cocktails & Chocolate--and You Can, Too!* Beachbody LLC, 2020.

7   "Idol Definition & Meaning." *Merriam-Webster*, www.merriam-webster.com/dictionary/idol.

8   DiNicolantonio, James Dr. (@drjamesdinic). "Obesity Statistics." *Instagram*, 22 February 2023, https://www.instagram.com/drjamesdinic.